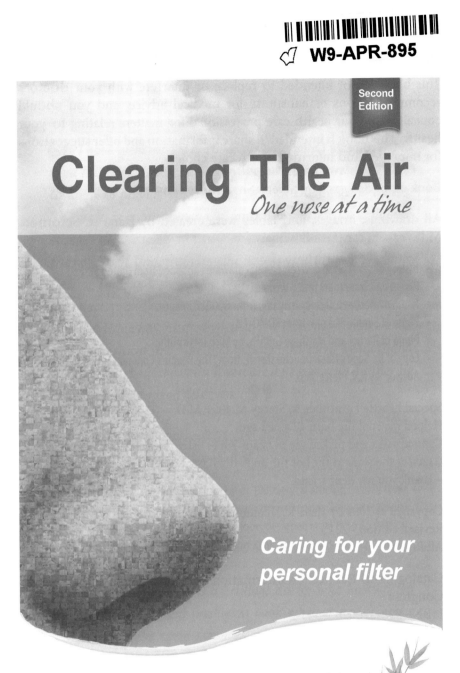

Second Edition

Clearing The Air
One nose at a time

*Caring for your
personal filter*

By Hana R. Solomon, M.D., Pediatrician

❝ *Congratulations on a wonderful update with the 2nd edition of your book, Cleaning the Air, One Nose at a Time!*

This is the book that I wish I had written myself! It encompasses all of the ailments that are related to the nose. As you clearly understand, the nose is central to all respiratory ailments, from otitis, to rhinitis, sinusitis, asthma, bronchitis, and even bad breath. And, the nose even plays an important role in lower respiratory infections like pneumonia, and the complications of Cystic fibrosis.

This is a wonderful collection of useful information, and should be the Owner's Manual for anyone with a nose! **❞**

Russell Faust, MD, PhD, FAAP, ABIHM (aka boogordoctor, at boogordoctor.com)
CEO, Sacred Herbals, LLC (sacredherbals.com)

❝ *Being a family physician with chronic allergies, vasomotor rhinitis, and sinus issues, I know the nose inside and out. I know how great an effect the nose has on our overall health and sense of well being. I am so grateful for Dr. Hana's book because it explains the anatomy, function, and care of the nose in easy to understand terms that I can share with my patients. In my practice I stress patient empowerment and preventive medicine, and I plan to enthusiastically recommend her well written and complete book to anyone with a nose!* **❞**

Stacey Kerr, M.D., Board Certified Family Physician
and author of Homebirth in the Hospital

66 *Nasal saline irrigation is a simple, scientifically proven method for preventing and treating so many respiratory health problems. It has been a breakthrough for my patients with recurrent sinus infections, nasal congestion, asthma and colds. Every day I teach people to incorporate this time-honored and effective technique into their daily health program. Clearing the Air One Nose at a Time is a must-read for every doctor who sees patients and every patient with a nose!* 99

Jane Murray, M.D., Board Certified in Family Medicine and Holistic Medicine
Medical Director, Sastun Center of Integrative Health Care, Overland Park, KS

66 *In an easy to understand fashion, Dr. Hana's book clearly outlines many of the concepts involved with the care of the ears, nose and throat. This book places Dr. Hana as the expert in the science of nasal washing, and it should be required reading for anyone with nasal and sinus problems. It is time that nasal washing be used as a front line treatment for nasal and sinus complaints as well as for prevention.* 99

Kelvin Walls, M.D.
Board Certified Ears, Nose and Throat Specialist and American Academy of
Otolaryngology-Head & Neck Surgery Member

66 *I have been using a nose washing system for two years and I swear by it, and after reading Dr. Solomon's book I now know why it works.* 99

Bill Wax, Program Director and show host of
Sirius/XM Satellite Radio's B.B. King's Bluesville

Dedication

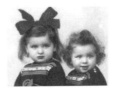

This book is dedicated to those who will never be able read this book; these words and ideas belong to them.

To all those who taught me and to all who held my hand.

To my grandmother Sabta, who demonstrated how to really survive. She survived the Holocaust with all four children intact and taught me to be strong no matter the obstacles.

To my mother Elza Drapacz whose wisdom, compassion, and never-ending faith allowed me the freedom to find *me*. She taught me how to be appreciative of what I have. If I came home with a cut on my eye, she would say "Thank God it wasn't both eyes."

To my children Josh, Vera, Rachel, and Marcus who accept my still-youthful dreams and who are each living their own dreams.

To all the babies in my life - Sophia, Eliot, Ava, Jordan, and Benjamin - who remind us that sweet life goes on.

To my late sister Jeannie, who showed me how to taste all the spices that life offers, who danced to her own music, and who helped me grow up.

To Jeannie's children, whom I adore and hold as dear to my heart as my own: Solomon, David, Josh, and Michelle.

To my late father who showed me how to have fun and taught me the value of spirit, guts and artistic expression.

To my late grandfather Marcus Drapacz, my dear 'Sabba', a sweet and tender soul. He taught me tolerance and acceptance. Sabba traveled to Missouri in his 80's while speaking no English, barely able to get around, just so he could share my communal family experience on The Farm.

To my lifelong best friend and endless supporter, no matter how outlandish my current dream may be, my husband George.

This book is dedicated to all those who struggle with their noses and to those whom I hope will learn to appreciate that wonderful filter.

Finally, this book is dedicated to all those who have yet to find their voice.

Dr. Hana

Hana R. Solomon, M.D., Pediatrician
Columbia, Missouri

Contents

Introduction 1

How to Use This Book 7

PART I: EVERYBODY HAS A NOSE

CHAPTER 1   Lay of the Land—Overview of the Nose............................ 13

Primary Function of the Nose: Defend, Protect and Shield *15*

The Magic of Mucus *16*

Mucus and Its Many Colors: Help, My Mucus Is Green! *18*

The Cilia Sweep *19*

Smell and Taste *21*

Moods *23*

Sexuality *23*

Other Uses for Your Nose *24*

Sinuses— What Are They and Why Do We Have Them? *25*

As The Nose Goes, the Ears Follow *29*

The Eyes Have It—An Intimate Connection with the Nose *32*

Facts: It's All Connected *33*

CHAPTER 2   Paying Through the Nose—The Cost of Nasal Woes.......... 35

CHAPTER 23 Medications.. 39

Medications and Additives for the Nose: Used, Misused, Abused *39*

Nasal Medications, Preservatives and Additives *40*

Nasal Spray Addiction: Rhinitis Medicamentosa (RM) *40*

Decongestants *41*

Antihistamines *42*

Other Medications *44*

PART II: KEEPING THE FILTER CLEAN

CHAPTER 4   Nasal Washing — Dilution Is the Solution to the Pollution . 51

What's That Smog in the Air? *51*

The History of Nasal Irrigation *55*

The Evolution of Medical Nasal Devices *58*

**CHAPTER 5   The Ins and Outs of Nasal Washing —
Taking Care of Your Great Defender.. 61**

Hypertonic Nasal Wash Solution *68*

Isotonic Nasal Wash Solution *69*

Hypotonic Nasal Wash Solution *70*

Buffering, pH and Acidity 71
Additives for Your Nose Wash Solution?.................................76
Xylitol, Baby Shampoo and Biofilms, Antibiotics / Antifungal
Agents, Hydrogen peroxide, Manuka Honey, Berberine
Botanicals, Quercetin, Grapefruit seed extract, Aromatherapy
and Essential Oils, Colloidal Silver, Silver Nitrate ....77 - 83
Nose Wash Style — So Many Choices! How to Choose?............84
The Importance of Head Position 85
Consider the Volume 87
Technique and Style 87
A Comfortable Habit...90
All in One Place: Common Nose Washing Systems 91
Nasal Irrigation Systems...94
The Dangers of Neti Pot Use—Fact or Fiction?......................96

CHAPTER 6   Dr. Hana's Nasopure **99**
The Nasopure Effect... 100
Salt. Is it Kosher? Does it matter?.. 104
Nasopure Studied for Effectiveness 104
Detailed Instructions on Using the Nasopure System........... 105
Possible Side Effects of Nasal Washing................................. 110

PART III: EVERYBODY HAS A NOSE

CHAPTER 7   Infants and Babies Need Clean Noses 121

CHAPTER 8   Children... 127
Kids and Colds - The Seemingly Endless Connection............. 127
Children and Ears 128
School Days 132
Teaching Your Child to Wash 135
How to Teach Your Two to Three-Year-Old Toddler to Wash.................. 136
How to Teach Your Four to Six-Year-Old to Wash 138
How to Teach Your Seven to Nine-Year-Old to Wash 139
Blow, Blow, Blow Your Nose Gently Now, Don't Scream 140
What If Your Preschool Child Is Scared of Water?................. 141

CHAPTER 9   Just for Women.. 147
Pregnancy and Hormones... 147
Women and Heart Disease: Is Air Pollution a Factor?........... 150

CHAPTER 10 The Seasoned Schnozz 151

CHAPTER 11 When Your Defense Is Down 157

Viral Infections 157
The Common Cold 160
Reminders When You Have a Cold.................................... 163
Sinus Problems and Bacterial Infections 170
Fungal Sinusitis 178
Allergies and Hay Fever 181
Saline Irrigation and Allergic Rhinitis............................... 184
Sore Throats: "My Throat Is Killing Me".......................... 188
The Scoop on Strep 190
Post-Nasal Drip 192
Constant Runny Nose (Vasomotor Rhinitis) 194
Cough, Cough, Cough.. 195
Asthma: Inflammation of the Airways 201
Sleep and Breathing Problems —More Serious Than You May Think ... 206
Vocal Cord Dysfunction (VCD) 209
Ears and Hearing Problems 209
Bad Breath (Halitosis).. 213
Nose Bleeds (Epistaxis) 214
Nasal Polyps 216
Deviated Nasal Septum... 219
Decreased or Absence of Smell (Anosmia) and Taste (Ageusia)............ 221
Cystic Fibrosis.. 224
Resistant Bacteria 228

CHAPTER 12 Normal Life Needs................................... 231
Can't I Just Buy an Air Filter? 231
Professional Voices 233
Military.. 237
Travelers 238
Smokers 240
Living and Working in Polluted Environments 240
Athletes and Sports Enthusiasts.. 243
Bicycles and Motorcycles.. 244
Golfers.. 246
Hikers, Campers and Gardeners 248
Scuba Divers... 248

Conclusion   251
About the Author.. 253
References   255
Index   257

Introduction

 Let's talk about your nose.

Let's talk about your kids' noses and your partner's nose and your grandparents' noses and your friends' noses.

In fact, let's talk about *everyone's* nose, because I know noses and what I know can help you.

Why do I care so much about the nose? Why should you care?

We have ignored the nose for far too long. The nose is more than just a bump in the middle of your face or a place for your sunglasses to rest. It is a part of your body that communicates with your outer world. It allows babies to continuously suckle on their mother's breast while easily breathing. The nose has the power to change your entire consciousness and mood in a single second - just expose your nose to a skunk. Or take a whiff of a rose.

The nose is our gatekeeper, our personal filter, and our great defender.

And when a nose fails in some fashion it affects the ears, sinuses, throat, appetite, and disposition. A dysfunctional nose can cause headaches, snoring, coughing and asthma, among other more serious conditions.

I know noses. Trust me, I'm a doctor. Shucks, as a pediatrician for over 20 years, I consulted with innumerable patients whose noses were snotty, congested, itchy, drippy, plugged, dry, sneezy, bloody, and overmedicated. My common-sense first response has always been, "Wash it first."

I guess you could say I was raised to have an "arms-length" relationship with the medical community.

It all began with my mother and my Sabta back in Brooklyn during the 1950s. My grandmother always insisted on chicken soup for any illness.

Despite her petite stature, she would declare, in her native tongue: "Eat. It's good for you!" On the other hand, I'm certain I never heard Sabta say, "Take this medicine. It'll make you better." As a child, I do not recall ever being given a pill for anything, *ever*. Only once did my doctor insist on a medication, a shot no less, when I was really ill.

During the 70s, in my early twenties, I joined a group whose lofty goal was to change the world by living off the Earth and leaving a tiny carbon footprint. There I found inner peace by growing organic food and preserving as much as possible for those long cold winters out on The Farm. I centered my life on beans, greens, meditation, and forgiveness. In this way, I was hoping to repair and change the world.

But the world was not changing fast enough and we were dirt poor. I could barely help myself, let alone anyone else. My teenage experience of volunteering as a candy striper in a Brooklyn hospital seeded my idea of being a doctor, but I lacked confidence. I had no role models to encourage me to pursue this outlandish notion. Me? A doctor? You must be joking! But somewhere, in the deepest part of me, I still wanted to be a doctor.

I dared not voice my dream. At least, not until my personal growth experience of living on the farm with beans, greens, and meditation fertilized my determination and strength.

When I was twenty-seven I left The Farm and began undergraduate studies with the goal of becoming a doctor. I completed four years of college in three years, and exactly three years after my exit off The Farm I started my first day of medical school as a single mom with two children.

The women in my family demonstrated for me, through their own lives, how to live as independent thinkers. My learning process was most certainly skewed by my life experiences, maturity and appreciation for the natural world. I was primarily interested in prevention and avoiding invasive medications and surgeries. I listened intently when professors taught me compassion and patient empowerment. The technical skills of surgical procedures, the nuances of x-ray procedures, and the minutiae of medical regulations were things I grasped quickly, and while I understood their importance I found them tedious. I knew through my own life experiences that the body is a miraculous organism, often able to heal itself if supported in the right environment.

Throughout medical school and residency I was blessed to receive training from a spectacular teacher of healing. As I listened to his lectures, I did not know the extent of his rare gift, but I did appreciate that he was special. Dr. Gullio Barbero, a pediatric gastroenterologist, would often take four hours or more to hear a family's story. Really, *four hours*. He taught all of us, both the medical students and the residents, that you must start at the beginning: the childhood of the parents. Then you must follow that timeline all the way to the current tummy ache; four hours was actually the *abridged* version. He demonstrated how this was the first step to understanding the way to heal compassionately. You must listen. The rest is easy.

Another remarkable teacher was Dr. David Parsons, an ear, nose and throat surgeon. His general message was "First, do no harm." This is, of course, part of the Hippocratic Oath, which all doctors take upon graduating from medical school. Dr. Parsons' specialties were sinus surgery, ear tube placements, tonsillectomies and adenoidectomies. However, his message was, "Never perform surgery on a child if it can be avoided." He shared the notion that irrigation of the nose makes sense *before* a patient goes into the operating room. He taught that washing could even *prevent* a trip to the operating room.

I took this advice to heart.

During the decades since completing my medical training I have learned much about the nose. For years I shared a clinic with my husband who is a family physician, so I have seen my share of adult issues in the nose, sinus, ears and lungs. Let's face it: I developed into the "snotty nose" expert. I studied, reviewed, discussed and listened to my patients and found I often encouraged nose washing as a way to avoid or reduce the need for medications. I also reviewed published scientific literature regarding nasal irrigation, and I found enormous support for this simple idea. More importantly, I asked every one of my patients to tell me about their experiences with nasal washing. Then I compared this feedback with the formal studies published in the medical literature.

Unfortunately, for over fifteen years, the majority of my colleagues just didn't get it. They were not incorporating nasal washing into their practices.

My patients confirmed what I witnessed to be true: those who washed their nose daily came to see me less often. Those who washed daily used fewer medications. Those who washed saved lots of money. Those who washed slept better, snored less, and experienced fewer asthma episodes.

A long time ago, we learned that if we brush our teeth daily, we prevent cavities. So now we brush. We know that all sorts of filters, whether for the car, the clothes dryer, the home heating and cooling system … all work better if kept clean. Why not clean the body's filter?

This makes sense to me. It has made sense to Buddhist monks for millennia. Jala Neti is the ancient practice of nasal washing performed as a daily hygiene routine in the eastern world. Even our grandmothers knew that moisture in the nose makes sense. Have you ever sniffed salt water when you had a cold? Remember placing your head over a steamy pot or in the warm shower when you were ill? Ever used a humidifier? How about that clean feeling after an ocean swim? Washing the nose uses a similar principle, but *far more easily, efficiently, and effectively.*

The question for me was: why did so many patients *not* follow my simple suggestion? Every parent knows that when a child falls and scrapes a knee, the wound is first washed, and *then* an antibiotic ointment is applied, if necessary. What was preventing more of my patients from incorporating nasal cleansing as a daily hygiene practice?

There were many hurdles. Convenience was a big hurdle. Availability was another one. The "yuck" factor was a common obstacle. "You want me to do what? And where?!" was a familiar response from patients. Because of this, I began my journey of finding the ideal nose washing system for my patients.

I am a medical doctor who thinks like a mom. I have been teaching nasal washing since long before it was "cool." I was "green" before that was cool, too. I have witnessed as both a patient and a physician the value and effectiveness of a preventive, holistic, patient-empowered approach. As a pediatrician, I have seen thousands of snotty noses, ear infections, sinus issues and asthma episodes. And my focus has been on avoidance of medications whenever possible. First, "Do No Harm."

This book is not intended to be a comprehensive compilation of all the issues related to the nose, nor a medical reference book. It is, however, full of good information and common-sense knowledge which I believe might be helpful in your journey to learn more about your body's air filter and how it relates to your overall health.

In life, as in medicine, nothing is absolute; everything is relative. The more you know, the better able you are to make choices that fit into your life. I share this with you so you can become empowered.

One more thing, and let's get this straight: we are talking about snot, goobers, boogers and mucus here, so please, do not be offended.

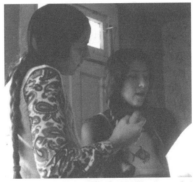

Stacey and Hana, young mothers studying pediatrics while cleaning house

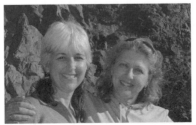

Stacey Marie Kerr M.D., Hana R. Solomon, M.D.

How to Use This Book

This book is for you if:

You have a nose,

You are the parent of sick and snotty-nosed kids,

You are a health care provider,

You live or work in a polluted environment, or

You want to have fewer problems with your nose, you want to use less medication and visit the doctor less often.

Part I: Everybody Has a Nose, is an overview for everyone who has a nose. You will find detailed, scientific explanations of the anatomy, functions and dysfunctions of the nose and related organs in this section. I feel it's important that you become familiar with the basics. Remember, the more you know, the better equipped you are to make decisions. You may find the master diagrams helpful.

Part II: Keeping the Filter Clean, is about how to clean your nose and how to keep this important filter working well for you.

Part III: Every Nose is Special, covers specific conditions for various groups of people. Choose the sections that apply to you.

Full disclosure: This book is a plea, a pitch, an argument, an appeal, even a nag, in favor of daily nose washing. It is not an endorsement for Nasopure, a product that I have developed and patented. I do want to be clear: it is impossible for me to discuss and present the most up-to-date comprehensive information on nasal washing without mentioning Nasopure, because it is the system I know well through years of clinical experience. There are no paid endorsements in this book; every shared experience has been freely given by grateful nose washers. I hope that my full and complete disclosure here "clears the air" and explains any perceived product endorsement you might find in this book.

What is far more important is this: daily washing will keep your nasal passages and sinuses clean, clear, and healthy. Allergists, family doctors, pediatricians, ear, nose and throat surgeons, naturopathic physicians and nurse practitioners all agree that nasal washing is safe and effective. You will hear from many of these experts as you read this book. What might be even more meaningful is that tens of thousands of people agree that nose washing, done correctly, feels good and refreshing and actually improves the quality of their lives. I truly don't care what you use to wash, as long as *you use something every day to keep your nose clean and healthy.*

Welcome to our knowledge place.

Master Diagram 1

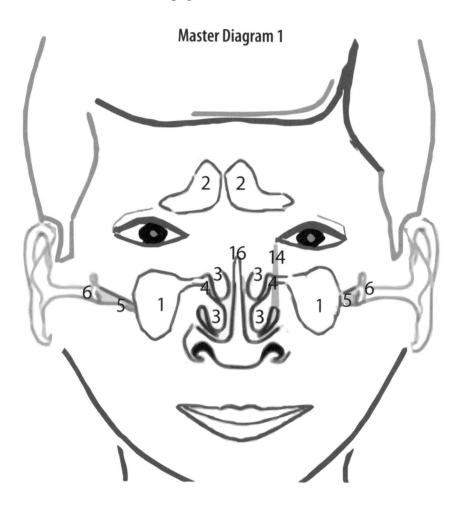

Master Diagram 2

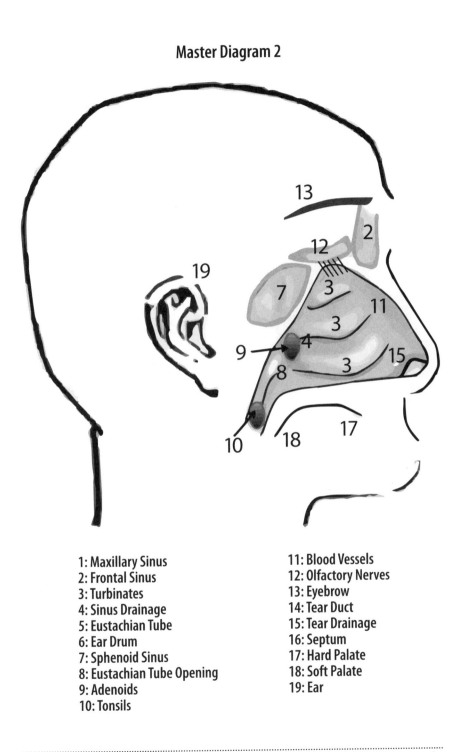

1: Maxillary Sinus
2: Frontal Sinus
3: Turbinates
4: Sinus Drainage
5: Eustachian Tube
6: Ear Drum
7: Sphenoid Sinus
8: Eustachian Tube Opening
9: Adenoids
10: Tonsils

11: Blood Vessels
12: Olfactory Nerves
13: Eyebrow
14: Tear Duct
15: Tear Drainage
16: Septum
17: Hard Palate
18: Soft Palate
19: Ear

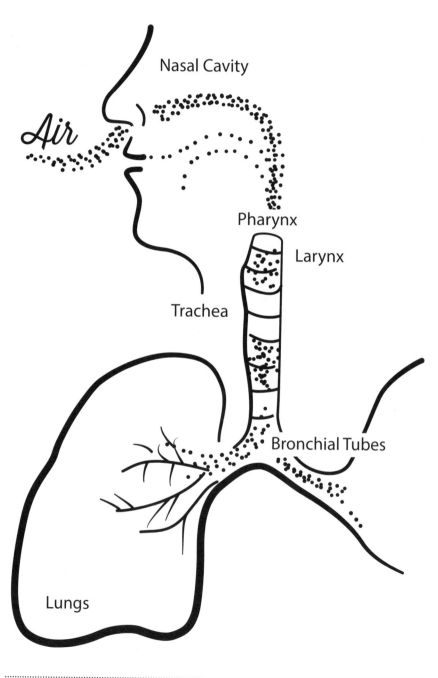

Nasal Cavity

Air

Pharynx

Larynx

Trachea

Bronchial Tubes

Lungs

Part I

Everybody Has a Nose

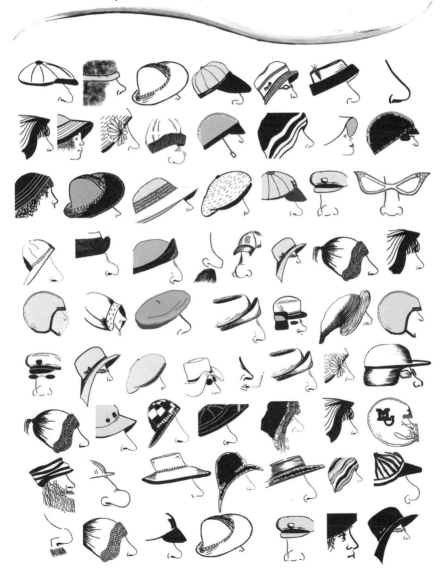

Chapter 1

Lay of the Land—
Overview of the Nose

I have always practiced medicine with a basic premise: my patients and I are a team. I acknowledge their values, preferences, and experiences so that I can understand their needs. I then share what I know, both book and clinical knowledge. A patient will ultimately make his or her own best choice; being an informed consumer makes the most sense for ideal health. With this in mind, I'd like to share my knowledge of the nose and all related structures so you can choose what works for you. This book is not intended to be comprehensive, but will be thorough as it relates to nasal health. All the scientific minutiae one wishes to learn can be found in other publications and in references listed in this book.

The nose is an elegant structure, beautifully designed for essential and life-supporting functions. It is not simply an air-intake port. When the nose works well, it filters, warms and humidifies the air we breathe (10,000 liters each day) - no small task in today's environment. The nose is the first major defense the human body has to protect us from our polluted world. For example, a sneeze is the body's initial protection to expel something considered noxious or even dangerous.

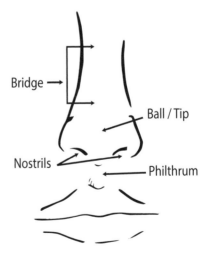

Without this filtering mechanism, millions of impurities would be allowed into our fragile lung tissues, wreaking havoc and damaging the gas-exchanging membranes deep within our chests. Without the oxygen-humidifying mechanism in our nose, our throat and airways would be dry and irritated all the time, and our moist lungs would dry out like a sponge left in the sun.

What we see of the nose is simply its outer covering and the two intake portals. The outer shape creates the illusion that the nose goes *up*. However, the nose really goes straight back into your head. The medical providers who specialize in the nose can safely insert a probe into your

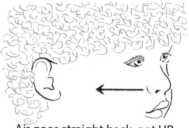
Air goes straight back, not UP

nose, directed straight back without any discomfort, yet a probe cannot be inserted upward more than a fraction of an inch. This common misconception has implications you will learn about as you read on. Remember, the nasal passages tunnel straight back!

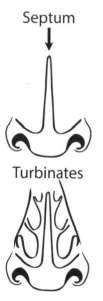
Septum

Turbinates

Even when we are forced to breathe through our mouths, our bodies attempt to moisturize the incoming air by using the tongue as a makeshift humidifier. The healthy and clear nose is a much more efficient and effective air conditioner than the tongue. The nose needs to expose a maximum amount of its intake to the air conditioning apparatus, so it is divided into two wind tunnels *(nostrils)* separated by a thin layer of cartilage called the *septum*.

The septum divides only the front of the nose into two nostrils - the back of the nose is a single chamber. Each nostril is designed to increase surface area with three rolls of tissue *(turbinates)* on each side. The air we inhale passes over these turbinates, picking up moisture along the way.

As the air swirls and spins, it passes across tiny hairs built into the lining of the nose. These hairs act as filters, capturing particles before they can reach the tender lungs and cause damage. Hairs just inside the nostril are coarse, but the ones further back are small and almost microscopic. When these tiny hairs *(cilia)* are allowed to move freely, and are not gummed up by debris and mucus, they do an excellent job of cleaning the air we breathe and protecting our lungs.

Sometimes an irritant gets caught, either on those folds of tissues called turbinates, or in the cilia. When this happens, we might sneeze or our nose may itch. More mucus is produced and our nose lining swells, resulting in the familiar congested feeling. All of these reactions are really part of the body's design to protect itself from impurities. We can help the nose filter more effectively by washing this air conditioning system. Flushing the filter clean is an effective way to help our nose do its job in today's complex and sometimes unclean environment.

Primary Function of the Nose: Defend, Protect and Shield

There are many nasal irritants in our world: smoke (fires and cigarettes), allergens, pollution, infectious particles (virus, bacteria, fungus) and excessive mucus. Amazing things happen immediately after one is exposed to irritants.

First, those rolls of tissues *(turbinates)* swell. Increased mucus production occurs. The mucus gets thicker and stickier. The filtering hairs *(cilia)* become clogged. As a result, all the normal drainage systems fail to function. Excessive mucus drips down the throat. There is a decrease in our ability to smell, taste, or hear. We may notice increased sinus pressure, headaches, bad breath or decreased exercise tolerance. Symptoms of chronically obstructed drainage include fatigue, poor appetite, decreased ability to concentrate and even bloody noses.

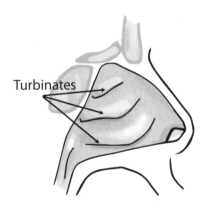
Turbinates

Irritants are not the only cause of nasal congestion. Air that is cold or dry can also cause congestion of your nasal passages. The congestion slows the airflow to ensure that your lungs receive warm and moist air. And while this reaction may help protect your lungs, the resulting congestion is not pleasant.

Nasal Air Flow

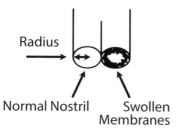

Radius

Normal Nostril   Swollen Membranes

The nasal opening, with its general rounded shape, follows basic laws of physics. Any decrease in the radius decreases the actual amount of airflow enormously. In practical terms, a tiny amount of swelling in the nasal passages can result in significant discomfort.

The turbinates' tissue folds increase surface area so more of the inhaled air can be conditioned. But what else is in the nose that allows it to act as such a great defender against irritants? Let's look at mucus and cilia.

The Magic of Mucus

Secreted by special cells, mucus is the substance that you know as "snot," "boogers," or "goobers" - terms that our children delight in saying. Nasal discharge, nasal drainage, rhinitis, sputum and phlegm are also terms used to describe this stuff.

But let's clear up the difference between *mucus* and *mucous*. Mucus is the stuff we know as nasal discharge. Mucous membranes are the actual lining of the nose and the sinuses. The mucous membranes secrete mucus.

Mucous membranes blanket the nose and other body parts. This membrane lining contains special *goblet cells* that produce mucus, a complex substance that keeps the nose and sinuses moist. We produce between one pint and one quart of mucus per day, thanks to goblet cells. That's two to four cups, or eight to sixteen ounces per day!

Certain proteins in the goblet cells determine the thickness, stickiness (viscosity), and stretchiness (elasticity) of the mucus. Mucus is usually very watery but it gets thicker and stickier when exposed to irritants such as allergens, infections and pollution. In addition, hydration, age, hormones and medications affect the consistency of mucus. Older people experience thicker and stickier mucus because of hormonal changes, as do pregnant women.

During cold weather, the nose hairs do not work as well to sweep the mucus towards the back of the throat and this explains why we often develop a runny nose when exposed to very cold temperatures. Mucus also thickens in cold weather. When an individual comes in from the cold, the mucus thins and begins to run before the cilia begin to work again.

Mucus traps irritants and protects our entire airway before being expelled. There are two layers in the mucous membrane lining of your nose. The outer layer is thick and rich with immune cells, antibodies and antibacterial proteins. This layer traps bacterial, viral, and particulate matter. The thinner, underlying layer enables the cilia to beat, their tips essentially grabbing the superficial layer and pushing it in the direction in which the cilia are beating, usually towards the back of the throat. Most normal mucus is swallowed and the trapped irritants are inactivated in the intestines (*gastrointestinal tract*) before leaving the body.

A problem occurs when mucus blocks the sinus or ear drainage openings. If the sinus opening (*osteomeatal complex*) becomes plugged we are at risk for infection or at the very least a sinus pressure headache. Similarly, if the ear drainage tube (*Eustachian tube*) gets clogged, ear pain, decreased hearing, infection, and other maladies can occur. When the normal flow of mucus is inhibited for any reason (*mucostasis*), dangerous bacterial, viral, or allergen particles can remain on cell surfaces long enough to penetrate the body's defense system.

Excess draining down the throat is called *post-nasal drip*. This can cause a cough, a change in voice quality or a sore throat. Mucus is naturally acidic and can burn the throat if allowed to stagnate there. Hence the complaint, "I woke up with a sore throat" is often a result of mucus drainage during sleep. Enough mucus and swelling can also cause a decreased sense of smell and taste.

Mucus and Its Many Colors:
Help, My Mucus Is Green!

In general, mucus is clear, thin, watery and even slimy. If infected with viral, bacterial or fungal particles, mucus normally changes to colors that can include white, yellow, green, brown, grey, or even blood-tinged. Discolored mucus can often have an offensive odor.

Many people assume that if their mucus is clear or white they are not infected, but if the mucus is yellow or green they require an antibiotic. This is not true. In fact, when one has a common cold the mucus progresses from clear to white to yellow to green and sometimes grey or brown and then clears again, all within seven to ten days. If one has persistent (more than three to five days) yellow or green discharge, then a bacterial infection *may* be present. We now know that even if a bacterial infection is suspected, a good flushing three to four times a day may prevent the need for medications. Only about 20% of bacterial sinusitis cases actually require antibiotics. Yes! Eighty percent of the time antibiotics are not needed!

This is also true for inner ear infections. NOTE: The antibiotic may treat the infection but will not address the original cause of the unhealthy environment.

People with asthma experience excess mucus production as part of the asthma inflammatory reaction, particularly in the bronchial tubes but also in the nasal cavity. This mucus is usually white and frothy and blocks or clogs the airways which in turn causes chest tightness, coughing, and wheezing.

Mucus Serves As a Frontline Defense

- Filters and moisturizes our air.
- Traps inhaled irritants (molds, pollen, dust mites, animal dander, smoke, ash, pollution).
- Protects against bacterial or viral invasion.
- Contains bacteria-fighting substances, including natural antibodies.
- Moistens food, making it easier to swallow and pass through the intestine.
- Smoothes the airway's linings and traps foreign substances before they invade the lower respiratory system.

The Cilia Sweep

Remember the little hairs (*cilia*) that blanket the inside of the nose and the sinuses? These are tiny projections which move in a wave-like pattern to transport mucus and all filtered material from the nose. Most mucus and debris is swallowed, spit out, or physically removed by blowing the nose.

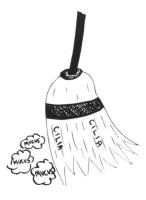

I like to think of cilia as a broom because they function to sweep the mucus outward. The sinuses in their healthy state are relatively empty, thanks to the constant sweeping of the mucus against gravity. The cilia work in unison to move the mucus through the drainage openings (*ostia*). The mucus is drained into the nasal cavity where it then exits out of the nose or onto the back of the throat. When cilia do not function properly due to infection, smoking, or a congenital problem (rare), mucus is not properly cleared. Infection then becomes a self-perpetuating process during which the infected mucus interferes with the normal sweeping process of the cilia, and this in turn prevents proper clearance of the mucus.

Cilia filter and mobilize...
debris, mucus, irritants, pollen, dust particles, virus, bacteria.

Mucus traps...
particles and moistens membranes.

Sinus and Ear Openings (ostia)...
allow normal mucus to drain from sinuses and ear cavities.

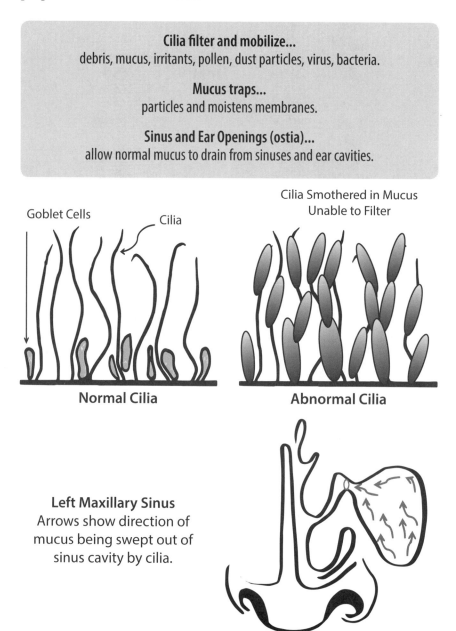

Cilia Smothered in Mucus
Unable to Filter

Goblet Cells

Cilia

Normal Cilia

Abnormal Cilia

Left Maxillary Sinus
Arrows show direction of mucus being swept out of sinus cavity by cilia.

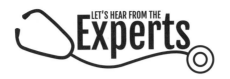

One of the nose's major tasks is to filter the air before it enters the lungs. Dust, smoke, dander, microorganisms and pollen contaminate the air at times and the small particles are caught by the mucus of the nose. Many of these are quite irritating to the nose. The nose normally protects itself with a mucus blanket that is moved by microscopic hair-tipped cells to the back of the nose where it is swallowed and the stomach juices are fairly effective in destroying these agents. When the nose is inflamed, it is not able to remove the noxious agents. Inflammation worsens the longer these agents remain in the nose.

Nasal irrigation with saline is effective in removing these noxious agents. Nasal saline solutions are available to spray as a mist which moisturizes the nose, but I believe that large volume irrigation is required to remove the harmful agents from the nose.

Jerry Templer, MD
Professor of Otolaryngology
University Of Missouri-Columbia School of Medicine

Smell and Taste

Both of these senses are directly related to the health of the nose.

Smell (*Olfactory system*)

What would life be like without the ability to smell? The term *anosmia* means lack of or decreased sense of smell.

The olfactory nerve cells with their special ends, called *olfactory receptors*, are located at the upper area of each nasal cavity. This is why we sniff to increase the ability to smell subtleties. The average nasal cavity contains more than 100 million olfactory neurons. In newborns, the nerve endings are a compacted sheet, but in children and adults, these tissues become less dense and interwoven. As humans age, the number of olfactory neurons steadily decreases.

The sense of smell is initiated by airborne chemicals that enter the nasal cavity in circular currents of air movement. These chemicals stimulate our olfactory nerves. The response to an odor is directly related to the sniff's duration, volume and velocity. The ability to smell can be compromised if the olfactory receptors are covered in mucoid debris.

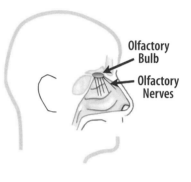

Olfactory Bulb

Olfactory Nerves

Taste (*Gustatory system*)

Considered the fifth sense, taste is mostly the smell of food in the mouth. *Ageusia* refers to a lack of or reduced ability to taste sweet, sour, bitter or salty substances.

Taste buds are tiny projections embedded in the tongue; a single taste bud can respond to multiple types of tastes. Taste buds cover the tongue, but are also located on the soft palate, epiglottis, larynx, and pharynx. There are eight to ten thousand taste buds in the human mouth.

Certain tastes are appreciated by anatomical locations. For example, sweetness is most readily detected at the tip of the tongue, whereas salty taste is detected at the front and sides of the tongue. Sour tastes are along the sides and bitter sensations are appreciated at the back of the tongue.

In humans and many other vertebrates, the sense of taste works with the sense of smell in the brain's perception of flavor. The gustatory system is intertwined with the olfactory system - that is to say, smell and taste are very closely related. Anyone who cannot smell appreciates the fact that his or her food tastes differently or does not have any flavor at all. See *Loss of Smell and Taste* on page 221.

Moods

Smells and the ability of the nose to fully function can affect our mood. Remember the last time you were exposed to a foul odor? You immediately felt a disgust or distaste for the source. Remember the last time you smelled something romantically appealing? It can aid in creating a sensual experience, which leads to many normal and delightful life activities. Candles, perfumes and aromatherapy are all booming businesses, a clear indication of how odors affect our moods. I am certain you can relate to a past experience when you were exposed to a scent which evoked childhood memories.

Sexuality

The nose contains tissue that is identical to our sexual organs' erectile tissue. The turbinates inside the nose contain large collapsible pockets of blood called *venous sinusoids*. These sinusoids become engorged and swell in response to irritants, resulting in decreased airflow. When you are exposed to any irritant, the instantaneous reaction causes the typical congested nose. Have you ever walked into an environment that contains strong irritants? Your nose instantly swells and feels dried, stuffy, and blocked. *Immediately*. Like an erection.

In evolution, survival is based on the ability to smell. The concept of human pheromones, or sexual scents of attraction, has been debated and researched for years. Pheromones' existence in humans may be in dispute but if you think about it, how often have you been turned off just by someone's smell, or the reverse, turned on by a subtle perfume?

If you're looking for the mate of your dreams, pheromones may contribute to this attraction. Our body odors, perceived as pleasant and sexy to another person, are part of a highly selective process. Pay attention to those signals when looking for a mate!

There is still much to learn about these substances but we do know that the nose and sexual behavior are related.

Other Uses for Your Nose

 On a lighter note, rubbing noses with someone you really like just wouldn't be the same without a nose, would it? What non-Eskimos call "Eskimo kissing" is loosely based on a traditional greeting and form of expressing affection, usually between family members and loved ones.

Think how hard it would be to keep your glasses in front of your eyes, not to mention how sore your ears would get, if you didn't have a nose.

Functions of the Nose

- Filter the air we breathe
- Moisten the air we breathe
- Warm the air we breathe

Dr. Hana's
CLINICAL ● PEARLS

Ear pain? Look in the nose.

Loss of taste? Look in the nose.

Headache? Look in the nose.

Sore throat? Look in the nose.

Asthma poorly controlled? Look in the nose.

Snoring? Look in the nose.

Sinuses—
What Are They and Why Do We Have Them?

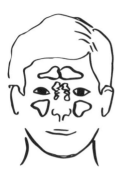

The sinuses are air-filled pockets within the skull, one pair on each side of the nose (the maxillary sinuses), one pair just between and above the eyebrows (the frontal sinuses), and two sets behind the nasal cavity (the ethmoids and sphenoids).

The function of the sinuses has been the subject of extensive research and we still have much to learn. What we do know is that the sinuses contribute to conditioning the air we breathe, give resonance to the voice, assist in absorbing shock, reduce the weight of the skull, and contribute to facial growth. If we did not have sinuses, our skulls would be too heavy to carry around; they lighten our load and influence our facial form.

The *osteomeatal complex* is the sinus drainage area, tucked between the lower two turbinates and emptying into the back of the throat. This important system of sinus openings collects mucus discharge from the various sinus cavities.

There is a phenomenon called *stagnation* that can occur at the osteomeatal complex - the main intersection of the drainage system. Stagnation occurs when the nose lining swells, blocking the osteomeatal complex and disrupting normal mucus clearance. This results in an unhealthy sinus environment. Clearance of the

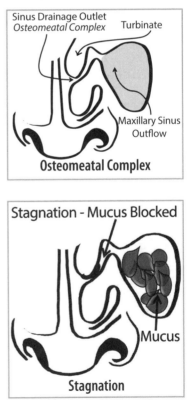

nose is accomplished when free-flowing secretions, open draining ports, and freely moving cilia have been restored.

The sinuses, like the nose, secrete mucus and contain cilia. Interestingly, the nose contains many more mucus-producing goblet cells than the sinuses, and thus produces more snot. Of the various sinus cavities, the maxillary sinus has the most goblet cells.

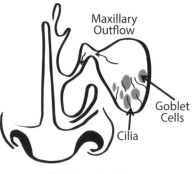

Maxillary Outflow

The cilia present in the sinuses work to move mucus in wave-like sweeps outward, toward the opening. Sinus cilia beat at a rate of 700-800 beats per minute and move mucus at a rate of 9 mm per minute. The movement of mucus is known as *mucociliary clearance*, or transit time. This clearance is vital since some sinuses drain via an opening at the top rather than the bottom, and the cilia must move mucus against gravity. It is interesting to note that hypertonic saline nasal irrigation has been shown to improve this transit time by 17% .

The sinuses drain into the osteomeatal complex and if clear, will drain normally. If obstructed by disease or normal body variations, the sinuses are unable to move mucus out and congestion begins. This crucial location requires cleansing without disrupting the natural balance.

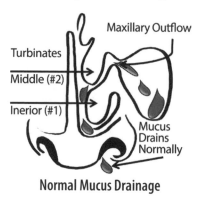

Normal Mucus Drainage

When all is working well, the sinuses are clear and empty of stagnant mucus.

Note: the exit *(maxillary outflow)* is small, located higher than the maxillary body and tucked between the turbinate folds. One can easily imagine how this becomes blocked due to colds, allergies, dried mucus and, as we will learn later, pregnancy.

As mentioned above, there are four pairs of sinuses in adults: *maxillary, frontal, ethmoid and sphenoid*. Babies are born with two of these sinus sets, the maxillary and the ethmoid. The remaining two sets develop during childhood, starting in the first year and expanding progressively until the child is in the early teens.

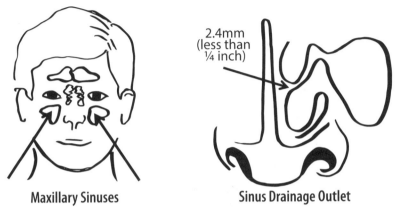

2.4mm (less than ¼ inch)

Maxillary Sinuses   **Sinus Drainage Outlet**

Maxillary Sinuses

The largest of the sinuses are the maxillary, one located in each cheek. Imagine a cave-like room with the only window at the very top of a wall, near the ceiling. This drainage port is higher than the body of the sinus. That means the cleansing sweep of the cilia must move *against* gravity.

The bony opening *(ostium)* size is very small, averaging 2.4 mm (a hair less than ¼ inch). The actual sinus opening is even narrower than the opening in the bone because the mucosa lining takes up space. Additionally, it is difficult for a doctor to see this tiny opening because it is hidden behind a bony protuberance. All of these factors contribute to a final sinus drainage port that is tiny and well hidden.

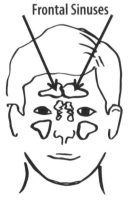

Frontal Sinuses

Frontal Sinuses

The frontal sinuses are located in the middle of the forehead. Unlike the maxillary cavities, they have their ostia at the bottom portion of the cavity, so they have gravity working for them. Accordingly, these sinuses are less likely to become infected.

Ethmoid Sinuses

The ethmoid sinuses are like sponges with tiny openings; this sponge is actually bone with many air cells. They are located at the roof of the nose, between the eyeballs. The bone is lightweight with approximately six to twelve small sinuses per side. The nerves, which allow us to smell the world around us, are located just below these sinuses. These sinuses drain indirectly into the osteomeatal complex.

Sphenoid Sinuses

Located directly behind the ethmoid sinuses, the sphenoid sinuses are near the middle of the skull. These can vary in both shape and size.

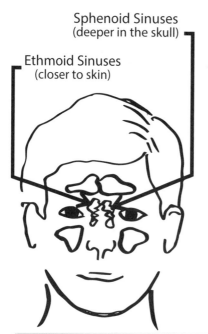

Sphenoid Sinuses
(deeper in the skull)

Ethmoid Sinuses
(closer to skin)

Often, the nasal septum can influence their contour. In fact, those with a deviated septum (a septum that is deviated a bit to one side) are more at risk of developing an infection in this particular cavity.

In general, a good washing of the nasal cavity is all that is needed to maintain a healthy environment for the tissues. Encouraging adequate drainage of the maxillary sinuses allows the natural process to proceed.

Three key elements necessary to maintain normal function of the nose and sinuses:

- Keep the cilia clean enough to keep on sweeping.
- Keep the sinus drainage port open and free to drain.
- Keep the mucus thin and free-flowing.

As The Nose Goes, the Ears Follow

Structure of the Ear

We can't look inside our own ears but we can sure feel what goes on in there! As you will soon learn, what goes on in the ears is intimately connected to the nose. Three distinct areas make up the human ear: the outer, the middle and the inner ear.

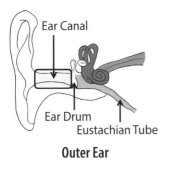

Outer Ear

The "ear canal" is part of the outer ear. This is the part we can see, the part that can get blocked with ear wax, and the part that captures sound from outside the body. The ear canal carries sound to a thin translucent membrane called the eardrum, or the *tympanic membrane*. It is the only portion a medical provider can easily observe in a clinic setting when evaluating a possible ear infection.

On the other side of the tympanic membrane is the middle ear, an air-filled chamber that contains the *ossicles* (three tiny bones all linked together). When the eardrum vibrates with sound coming from the ear canal, the ossicles pick up the vibrations and amplify them, carrying them to the inner ear. The inner ear translates those vibrations into electrical signals and sends them to the auditory nerve, which is connected to the brain. When these nerve impulses reach the brain, they're interpreted as sound.

How does this involve the nose? Well, there is a direct connection between the middle ear and the nose.

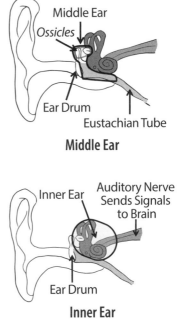

Middle Ear

Inner Ear

For sound vibrations to send the signals to the inner ear, the middle part of the ear must be ventilated, allowing the air pressure on either side of the tympanic membrane to equalize. The *Eustachian tube* is responsible for this ventilation. This tube begins in the middle ear and extends into the back of the upper throat, approximately at the same level as your nostrils. The portion of this tube nearest the eardrum is always open, protecting the middle ear. The end that drains into the back of the throat is normally closed. We open and close this part of the Eustachian tube when we chew and suck.

In adults, the Eustachian tube is approximately 35 mm long (1.38 inches). In children, it is significantly smaller and more difficult to drain for many reasons.

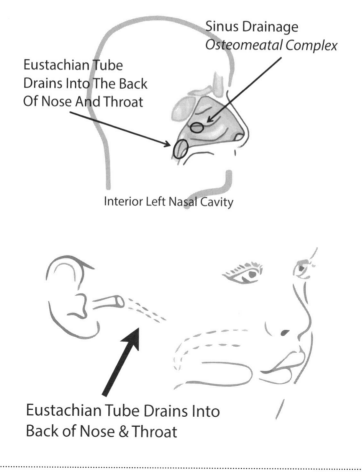

Sinus Drainage
Osteomeatal Complex

Eustachian Tube
Drains Into The Back
Of Nose And Throat

Interior Left Nasal Cavity

Eustachian Tube Drains Into
Back of Nose & Throat

Eustachian Tubes Differ Between Kids and Adults

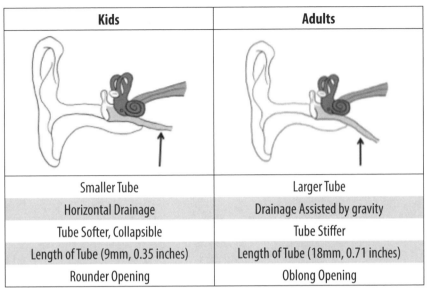

Kids	Adults
Smaller Tube	Larger Tube
Horizontal Drainage	Drainage Assisted by gravity
Tube Softer, Collapsible	Tube Stiffer
Length of Tube (9mm, 0.35 inches)	Length of Tube (18mm, 0.71 inches)
Rounder Opening	Oblong Opening

Who Cares When Your Eustachian Tube Does Not Work? You Do!

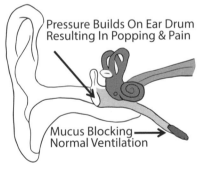

Pressure Builds On Ear Drum Resulting In Popping & Pain

Mucus Blocking Normal Ventilation

Eustachian Tube Dysfunction

The Eustachian tube drains mucus from the middle ear into the back of the throat. Upper airway infections or allergies can cause this tiny tube to become swollen, trapping bacteria and causing middle ear infections.

If air is bubbling up and mucus is flowing down and out into the throat, all is well. But for this to happen it is vital that the Eustachian tube remain open and free to drain. None of this can be accomplished if there is a mucus plug or if there is swelling, as both plugging and swelling prevent natural drainage.

Again, as the nose goes, the ears follow. Nasal health is critical for healthy ears.

The Eyes Have It—
An Intimate Connection with the Nose

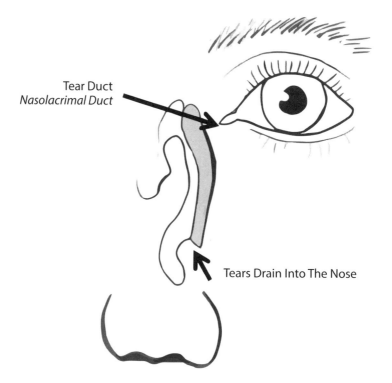

Tear Duct
Nasolacrimal Duct

Tears Drain Into The Nose

The tear duct *(nasolacrimal duct)* drains tears from the eyes and empties those tears under the lowest turbinate. This is why crying often results in nasal discharge. This also explains why nasal washing done incorrectly can push the solution up and out through the tear ducts.

This pathway may contribute to allergens entering the eyes, draining into the nose and causing allergic symptoms in the nose. There is also evidence that there may be backward *(retrograde)* flow from the nose back up into the eyes as well. For example, if you're wearing goggles but are exposed to outdoor pollen, you might develop itchy eyes. The pollen has entered the nose but because of the retrograde movement of the pollen, the eyes may itch. This is another example of how the individual parts of our facial anatomy are all connected.

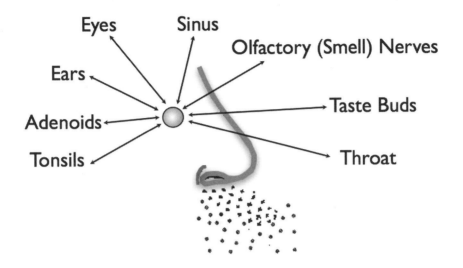

Eyes   Sinus

Olfactory (Smell) Nerves

Ears

Taste Buds

Adenoids

Tonsils

Throat

Facts: It's All Connected

- We breathe 10,000 liters of air per day through the nose.
- We produce one pint to one quart of mucus per day.
- We have 8-10,000 taste buds in the tongue.
- We have 100 million olfactory neurons.
- Cilia beat 700-800 beats per minute.
- Cilia beat 17% more effectively after washing with hypertonic saline.
- Normal pH of nasal mucus in adults is 5.5-6.5.
- Normal pH of nasal mucus in infants and children is 5.0-6.7.
- Best pH to foster excess mucus clearance is 6.9-9.5.
- Buffering with sodium bicarbonate improves the flow of mucus.
- Buffering is beneficial for both hypertonic and isotonic solutions.
- 60 million Americans suffer from allergies.
- 80% of infections of the ear and sinus will resolve with nasal washing alone.
- Sinus opening allowing mucus to drain is less than 1/4 inch.

Chapter 2

Paying Through the Nose—
The Cost of Nasal Woes

 The numbers are always changing, and they are *not* going down. Americans spend billions of dollars every year treating nasal, allergy, sinus, ear and asthma problems. The dollars spent are only part of the price tag. The cost in terms of time off work, away from school, sitting in a doctor's office and time spent feeling lousy is sky-high. How about time spent in the bathroom dealing with side effects of a medication? What about lost sleep, lack of focus, and impatience with family and co-workers?

If your nose isn't working properly you are losing time and money, as well as impacting your quality of life. You are, quite literally, paying through the nose. Consider these figures, just a sampling of the numbers illustrating the annual cost of nose woes:

- Billions of dollars spent on medicine and treatment for allergic rhinitis.
- Over 60 million Americans suffer from allergies and asthma each year.
- The majority of all antibiotic prescriptions are written to treat respiratory infections.
- Billions of dollars spent on the evaluation and treatment of ear infections.
- Quality of life is significantly reduced for those who suffer from hay fever.
- Asthma is the most common cause of school absenteeism due to chronic conditions.
- Billions of dollars spent to treat asthma per year.
- Children typically have two to nine viral respiratory illnesses per year.
- Those with allergic rhinitis often suffer from sinusitis as well as asthma.

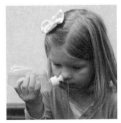 Okay, that's the bad news. The good news is you don't have to just suffer and spend money. You can do something to treat both the symptoms and the cause of these conditions. Let's see what an expert has to say about this situation.

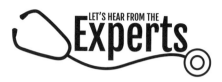

LET'S HEAR FROM THE
Experts

Marilyn James-Kracke, PhD is an associate professor of medical pharmacology and physiology. She teaches students preparing for careers in medicine, pharmacology and nursing; she is an expert on drugs! Her comments are based on her knowledge and personal experience.

Green Health Care (Prevention vs. Treatment)

Sick days cost the American economy billions per year. Lost work days stress both employers and employees. For those without substitutes to fill in, the thought of becoming ill invokes panic. To cope, they take extra precautions to stay well. I am one of those "solo" workers. I try to remain in tip-top shape by washing my nose twice daily.

I look upon my classroom as a microcosm of society because the pharmaceutical industry, health care industry and the population of this country affect topics we discuss. By allowing my imagination free rein, I can foresee industry, business, politics and finance benefiting if society assumes responsibility to reduce health care costs. Can nose washing help to cap these costs to improve the well-being of the nation? Permit me to expound on this topic.

Teachers benefit if children are not sneezing and coughing throughout class. Words of wisdom are more audible when there is no din of bark-bark-barkers, ha-ha-chachoo-ers and foghorn nose blowers. For daycare teachers, wiping noses of toddlers is an occupational hazard. School-aged children blow their own noses with variable degrees of success but still innocently spread airborne pathogens to menace everyone sharing the same air.

Since not breathing is not an option, flushing nasal germs down the drain to deplete their virulence makes more sense to reduce absenteeism. Do you remember substitute teachers who provided comic relief from an ogre-ish one? That was fun, but we learned little that day. It was a hardship when excellent teachers were absent or mothers collapsed in their line of duty. Working mothers should view nose washing as job and salary protection insurance.

Wherever people gather in confined spaces, they contract airborne illness. Planes, trains and buses are common perpetrators of germ warfare. How many people frugally save for a special vacation only to become sick as a dog while traveling? Think of nose washing as a form of travel insurance.

What are our alternatives? Should we wear face masks to prevent the spread of illness? We expect everyone to be vaccinated and toilet-trained, wash their hands, sneeze into tissues, brush their teeth and shower. Has the time come to add nose washing to standard daily hygiene?

What do I want to achieve? My intentions are to:
- Encourage the reduction of suffering and reduce the spread of illness to immune compromised patients like the elderly, infants and those undergoing chemotherapy.
- Make schools healthier learning environments.
- Make workplaces healthier and workforces more productive.
- Lower the cost of healthcare that is bankrupting the economy.

Americans must "save for a rainy day." Saving trees by reducing tissue use is a good idea too. Nasal washing reduces the need for certain drugs and hospital treatments. Given a choice between washing my nose for a minute a day and being congested perpetually all day I will wash my nose. We must demonstrate that nose washing does not cause drowning or even discomfort.

Marilyn James-Kracke, PhD
Associate Professor
Medical Pharmacology and Physiology
University of Missouri-Columbia

Chapter 3

Medications

Medications and Additives for the Nose: Used, Misused, Abused

No one would dispute the miracles of modern medicine: surgeries performed through minimal incisions, organ transplants, re-attachment of limbs, advances in chemotherapy, and the many lives antibiotics have saved. People would be best served if modern medicine would incorporate patient education, nutrition, and prevention, as well as complementary and alternative approaches. My personal perspective on medication use comes from this position: do I really need the drug? Are other options available? Would I give this to my child or to my mother? Is this one of those drugs currently approved by the government regulatory agencies that will, in time, be found to cause more harm than good?

There is no doubt the nose requires moisture for proper functioning. Things go wrong if the nose is dry. However, medications for nasal congestion, while occasionally necessary, only treat the targeted symptoms, not the root cause.

There are also risks to using nasal medications; some are easily abused. Let's look at a few common problematic medications.

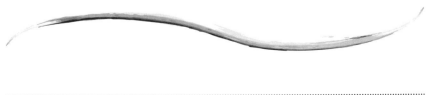

Nasal Medications, Preservatives and Additives

Nasal sprays are easy to use, but there is evidence that many of the preservatives and additives in some of the commercial nasal sprays can be harmful to the nose!

Some additives I like to avoid include benzyl alcohol, povidone, iodine, disodium ETA, edetate disodium, benzalkonium, thimerosal, merthiolate, monobasic sodium phosphate, dibasic sodium phosphate, potassium phosphate monobasic, phenylcarbinol and sodium silicoaluminate. Some of these can directly irritate the sensitive lining of the nose, and some can cause allergic reactions.

More warnings:

- Some topical nasal decongestants contain sulfites. Asthmatics may react to sulfites, and some of these reactions may be life threatening.

- Do not use nasal spray decongestants in children younger than two years old because these medications can interact with oral decongestants in cold medications.

- The nasal medications which contain benzalkonium chloride (BKC), a preservative that prevents the growth of microorganisms, can cause more rebound swelling than those that are BKC free. Thus, BKC may aggravate a condition known as Rhinitis Medicamentosa (RM, or nasal spray addiction, see below.)

Nasal Spray Addiction: *Rhinitis Medicamentosa (RM)*

Rhinitis Medicamentosa (RM) is a fancy name for physical addiction to a nasal spray. It is "rebound nasal congestion" caused directly by overuse and abuse of intranasal decongestants. These medications are vasoconstrictive, which means they close down blood vessels.

It continues to be unclear how decongestant nasal sprays cause the classic rebound swelling of RM, wherein congestion is worse after the effect of the spray wears off. What is clear is that the longer you use these sprays, the more often dosing is required to achieve the same benefit. In addition, when you try to quit using the medication, your nose reacts by becoming more swollen and congested than it was to begin with.

As a consequence of prolonged use of nasal decongestants, RM often leads to mucous membranes that are very abnormal in both appearance and function. They can appear very red, irritated and swollen with areas that easily bleed. Some reports suggest that the lining of the nose appears pale and anemic. The mucus is usually clear and minimal, unless an accompanying sinus infection is present. Others report profuse and thick mucus. In either case, the tissues are unhealthy and not able to function properly.

Because of the abuse of nasal decongestants, chronic sinusitis, chronic runny nose due to thinning of the nasal membranes, and permanent turbinate hyperplasia (development of excessive tissue inside the nose) can result. The cost of treating these side effects is considerably higher than the price of the medication.

Decongestants

 Many of us have reached for a decongestant when we are congested and stuffy. The active ingredient used in many over the counter decongestants, phenylephrine, is used to relieve nasal or sinus congestion caused by the common cold, sinusitis, hay fever and other respiratory irritants. This medicine and other similar drugs relieve stuffy noses, open nasal airways, and allow sinuses to drain. They are also used to relieve ear congestion caused by inflammation or infection.

This type of drug does decongest, but its use also comes with potential risks. Have you ever felt the jitters after taking this medicine? That's because it is a stimulant, with side effects which are potentially serious.

Serious reactions include heart arrhythmias and severe hypertension. More commonly, people who take this medication can experience insomnia, nausea, headaches, dizziness, nervousness, irritability, heart palpitations, weakness or tremors. There are specific warnings for women who are pregnant, for small children, and for people taking other medications. It is so easy to take a little tiny decongestant pill and then go on with your day. But before you do, inform yourself about what you are putting into your body.

So if a decongestant is worrisome, what choices do you have for that itchy, drippy, sneezy or stuffy nose? The safest, simplest option is a salty nose wash, which acts as a natural decongestant. Salty nose washes (hypertonic buffered saline) work to shrink swollen membranes naturally, without harmful side effects.

Antihistamines

What Are Antihistamines and How Do They Work?

 If you have allergies and are exposed to an irritant such as a pollen particle, a chemical called *histamine* is released from the body's cells. This chemical causes itching, sneezing, runny noses and watery eyes. Antihistamines prevent or reduce the symptoms caused by histamines. So antihistamines can treat *some* of the symptoms of allergies, colds and reactions to insect bites, stings, and poison ivy/oak.

Antihistamines cross into the brain and affect that portion of the brain which controls nausea and vomiting, so they are also used to treat motion sickness. In addition, some of the earlier first generation antihistamines cause sleepiness and can be effectively used to treat insomnia.

Side Effects of Antihistamines

There are two types of over-the-counter (OTC) antihistamines which can be purchased without a doctor's prescription: first generation and the newer, second generation antihistamines.

Best-known of the first generation OTC antihistamines is diphenhydramine (Benadryl). Others include brompheniramine (Dimetapp) and chlorpheniramine and dimenhydrinate (Dramamine).

These all tend to cause sedation but approximately 10-15% of people, particularly children, can have an opposite reaction and become stimulated (hyperactive, unable to sleep, or irritable). Only a trial of these medications will tell what kind of a responder you or your child may be.

When first-generation antihistamines make you feel sleepy, they adversely affect your ability to drive, operate machines, pay attention and think clearly. A 2000 study published in the *Annals of Internal Medicine* compared the effects of diphenhydramine and alcohol on driving response times. The conclusion stated "…diphenhydramine had a greater impact on driving than alcohol did." These first generation antihistamines can also cause dry mouth, dry eyes and thickened mucus, which may increase the risk of developing a sinus infection. Thick dry mucus creates a very effective block in sinus drainage openings, allowing infection and pain to take over.

Second generation antihistamines (Claritin, Allegra, Zyrtec) are *usually* non-sedating. However, each person is unique and some people do complain of sedating side effects with the newer products. These tend to have a longer lasting effect, up to 24 hours, unlike the first generation antihistamines which typically last four to six hours.

You should be aware that antihistamines are often combined with other drugs like decongestants, pain relievers, and mucus thinners (mucolytics). If you buy a pre-mixed combination, the risk of mixing two types of the same medication rises. Antihistamines can also interact with many other over-the-counter and prescription medications. This is particularly true in children and the elderly but it is not an uncommon event in the general population. Some antihistamines interact with other drugs by changing the way your body processes or clears the drug from your body, so beware before you mix antihistamines with sleeping pills, muscle relaxants or high blood pressure medications. In my practice, my preference and recommendation is to avoid the trap of convenience, and use only those individual medications which you clearly want or need.

Talk to your physician before taking first generation antihistamines if you have glaucoma, an enlarged prostate gland, asthma, emphysema, chronic bronchitis, thyroid disease, heart disease or high blood pressure. If you have liver or kidney disease, be careful and check with your doctor before using second generation antihistamines.

Other Medications

 There are scores of other medications available and often used for nasal woes. For the sake of completeness, I list some of the familiar ones here. Each medication has its place but also its potential ill effects. Just remember: stay informed and choose wisely.

- **Mucolytics** (Mucinex, generic guainefesin) are medications which thin mucus and other secretions - one of my favorites.

- **Cough suppressants** (codeine, dextromethorphan) inhibit the brain's reflex to cough - useful only on a very short term basis and usually best used at night to get some healing sleep. Recently, researchers have found that cough suppressants are no more effective in relieving children's nighttime coughs than placebos are, so pediatricians recommend avoiding their use in those younger than six years old. And remember: never "hide" a chronic cough unless you know the cause.

- **Nasal steroids** (Flonase, Nasonex, Rhinocort and others) inhibit the body's immune response to irritants. They have a long list of potential side effects, including the encouragement of fungal overgrowth, but can be helpful in low doses if applied to clean nasal membranes.

- **Nasal antihistamines** (Astelin) have few worrisome side effects. Applying this drug onto clean tissues is most effective.

- **Immune modulators** (cromolyn sodium, Singular) halt the allergic response in a different pathway compared to antihistamines. Treats the symptoms and the body's response to allergens, but does not address the root of the problem.

- **Antibiotics** attempt to treat the infection but do nothing for the original cause of the infection. Overuse is problematic, expensive and has risks. Often the majority of infections will resolve without the antibiotics.

- **Asthma medications** (inhaled anti-inflammatories, bronchial dilators) have numerous side effects, but can be lifesaving. There exists a wealth of knowledge addressing nasal and sinus problems, with nasal washing as a first line of defense, reducing the need for asthma medications.

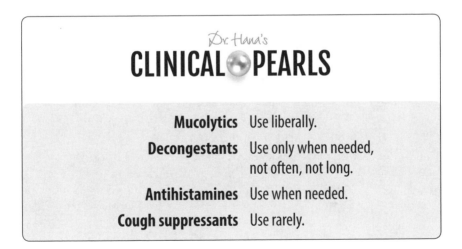

Dr. Hana's
CLINICAL PEARLS

Mucolytics	Use liberally.
Decongestants	Use only when needed, not often, not long.
Antihistamines	Use when needed.
Cough suppressants	Use rarely.

The Wall Street Journal published an article entitled "Waiting it Out: Antibiotics Are Unlikely to Help Sinusitis." Reporter Anna Wilde Mathews notes that antibiotics do little or no good in treating sinus infections and that, increasingly, doctors are turning to treatments that do not involve medications. This once again supports the recommendation that every sinus infection need not be treated with antibiotics.

A 2007 research study published in JAMA *(Journal of the American Medical Association)* reaches the same conclusion. The study reports that over-prescription of antibiotics can increase drug resistance. This leaves fewer options for treatment of serious infections. Dr. Ian Williamson, lead author of the study, notes "With a little bit of patience, the body will usually heal itself."

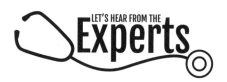
LET'S HEAR FROM THE Experts

Nasal steroids control symptoms caused by inflammation. The average benefit from this treatment is small but definite, and for some patients it may work especially well. Thus, a two-week therapeutic trial period is reasonable. If it is ineffective, it may work if tried again later. Although it can promote proliferation of yeasts and possibly other microbes, side effects are usually minor - perhaps mild nasal irritation or bleeding. Nasal steroids have a more definite benefit when there is nasal obstruction due to large adenoids. In adequate doses, a four to eight-week course can significantly reverse obstruction, sometimes enough to avoid surgery.

Michael Cooperstock, MD, MPH
Pediatric Infectious Disease
University of Missouri, Columbia, Medical Center
Avoided Decongestants

Avoiding Medications

....

❝ *About a year ago I really needed some pseudoephedrine-type decongestant and there was a long line at the pharmacy, so I ended up trying a nose wash. I have used it regularly and have come to like it a lot.* ❞

Laura T., Grand Forks, Minnesota

....

....

❝ *Nasal washing works. Everyone with allergies should do it. I don't buy sinus medicine anymore, and I don't have headaches.* ❞

Dana M., Louisville, Kentucky

....

....

❝ *It's been very common for me to have trouble breathing through my nose. I've almost always had at least one nostril blocked that will switch between nostrils throughout the day. Cat allergies, mold and dust have all taken a toll over the years. I recently had a deep nasal culture that shows an MRSA* staph infection residing in my sinuses. I've been using the Nasopure for about three weeks three times per day and have had some relief. Smells have been stronger at times and it has been easier to breathe from my nose. For example, there have been times over the past several weeks that I've been able to breathe through both nostrils. The results have been encouraging and I'm cautiously optimistic that continued use will get the staph.* ❞

Bruce S, Columbia, Missouri

....

* Methicillin-resistant Staphylococcus aureus (MRSA) infection is caused by a strain of staph bacteria that has become resistant to antibiotics commonly used to treat ordinary staph infections.

....

Part II

Keeping The Filter Clean

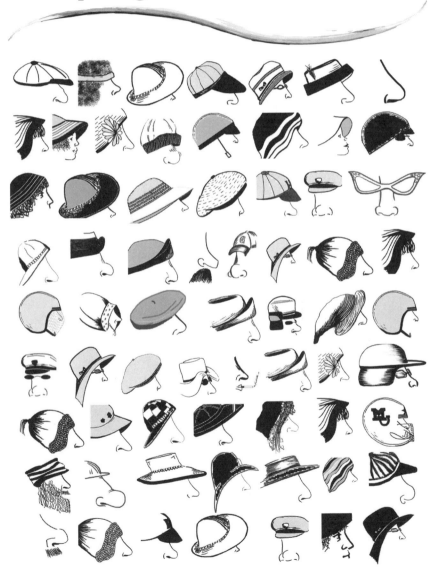

Chapter 4

Nasal Washing — Dilution Is the Solution to the Pollution

What's That Smog in the Air?

 Air pollution and how it affects our health continues to be studied. We know that the monetary costs of the resulting medical conditions are in the billions of dollars. Our quality of life costs are very high as well. Air pollution has both immediate and long-term effects.

Depending on your age, health status, and the air quality of your environment, the effects can vary. In addition, some people are just more sensitive to pollutants than others and, as in many other situations, both the very young and the elderly tend to be more at risk. Children are especially vulnerable to the effects of air pollution and experience ill effects at lower levels of pollution as compared to adults. It is also clear that kids in highly polluted environments experience higher rates of asthma, bronchitis and earaches.

If you have asthma, lung disease, allergies, Cystic Fibrosis, nasal polyps or heart issues, the effects are more significant. The ill effects of air pollution are directly proportionate to both time of exposure and the concentration of damaging chemicals in the air.

Short-term exposure can result in irritation to the eyes, nose and throat. It can cause chest tightness, cough and asthma flare-ups. Additional consequences can include an increase in upper respiratory infections, bronchitis, pneumonia, headaches, nausea, allergic reactions and emphysema exacerbations. If you participate in outdoor physical activities, symptoms are more noticeable and quick to occur.

Potential effects of long-term exposure to polluted air are chronic respiratory disease, lung cancer, and heart disease. There are also harmful effects to the brain, nerves, liver or kidneys and even negative effects on the immune system. Increased hospital admissions and premature deaths have been linked to prolonged exposure to pollution.

Although we are usually unable to see the pollution in the air we breathe, we can often smell it. But we get used to the smell of the air in our home communities so we cannot always know when we are at risk. Air pollution contains gases, droplets and particles and can be identified in both city and country air. Dust and smoke from transportation, construction and manufacturing all contribute to air pollution.

Another major contributor to air pollution is ground level ozone. This is created from engine and fuel gases and is at its worst on sunny, still and warm days. Do not confuse the harmful ground-level ozone with the protective ozone miles above the earth's surface which actually shields us from the sun's harmful radiation.

The government's Environmental Protection Agency (EPA) monitors and reports air quality in the United States. The EPA suggests measures you can take to protect your family on days when pollution is high:

- ✓ Stay indoors if possible.
- ✓ If you must go outside, limit outside activity to the early morning hours or wait until after sunset.
- ✓ Don't exercise or exert yourself outdoors. Exercise indoors.
- ✓ Wear masks.

This doesn't sound like too much fun and most likely you will still be going outside on days of high pollution. This makes it all the more important for you to keep your personal air filter in good working order. I suggest following these EPA guidelines and, upon returning from the polluted outdoors, wash your filter clean.

Nasal washing has finally become familiar to many consumers. Many years ago, when I introduced the idea of irrigation, the majority of my patients never even considered the idea of washing the inside of the nose.

At first, the suggestion was considered a bit on the edge. Today, most people have at least heard or read about this common-sense notion. I predict that eventually nasal washing will be part of most people's daily hygiene practice with wash systems in every bathroom and travel bag next to the toothbrush.

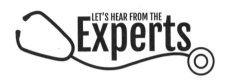

As population density and air pollution rise worldwide, the nose's natural function and burden of protecting the lungs and body from air pollution and germs may be overtaxed. With chronic sinus infections and allergies being widespread in the United States (NCHS, 1994), Europe and China, perhaps we are reaching a time in human and population development where a wide-spread practice of nasal hygiene might improve nasal and overall health.

Susan F. Rudy, MSN, CS-Nurse Practitioner, Washington, DC
Author, "Nuances of Nasal and Sinus Self-Help"

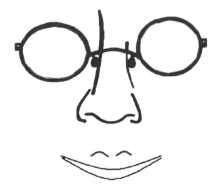

Why has nasal washing become so popular?

- Complementary, alternative and integrative medicine has boomed in popularity.

- Prevention is the new treatment.

- Less aggressive approach is green and good for the environment.

- Neti exposure from the "Oprah - Dr. Oz effect".

- Bacteria has developed resistance to antibiotics.

- Press coverage on the overuse of antibiotics.

- Drug recalls, such as cold preparations for kids.

- American Academy of Pediatrics' new guidelines regarding cold medicines, ear infections and overuse of antibiotics - warning doctors that they are prescribing these medications too often.

- Drug commercials with side effects of medications listed.

- Costs of medications.

- Internet information.

- Consumers are asking for advice and people want to know.
  - A Google search for "nasal irrigation" in 2000 resulted in fewer than 100,000 responses.
  - A Google search for "nasal irrigation" in 2005 resulted in 800,000 responses.
  - A Google search for "nose wash" in 2008 resulted in 11.4 million responses.
  - A Google search for 'nose wash' in 2013 resulted in over 250 million responses.

 I have lectured to medical doctors, respiratory therapists, nurse practitioners, and many other health care providers. I am frequently surprised by how often the question, "Isn't this the same as a saline nasal spray?" is asked, but when you think about it, it becomes rather obvious that a small spritz is quite different than a full flush. When you develop an infected wound, your medical provider's first step is to flush the wound with sterile water, not simply spray or mist it. Then, and only then, is further treatment even considered. I propose the same approach be taken with nasal, sinus and respiratory issues. It also occurs to me that the current focus of western medicine is all too often on treatment rather than prevention.

Why Do Medical Providers Need To Know About Nasal Washing?

- ✓ To be able to offer it as a treatment option for their patients.
- ✓ To become familiar with current nasal washing devices and various solution ingredients.
- ✓ To understand what system would be best for their patients.
- ✓ To become comfortable enough to incorporate nasal washing into the art of medicine.
- ✓ To understand the limitations of nasal washing.

The History of Nasal Irrigation

As early as 1882, western medical textbooks demonstrated nasal washing. Polish physician Alfred Laskiewicz, chief of Pozna Hospital Otolaryngology Department (1932-1939) described conservative treatments of nasal irrigation for general hygiene and for medical problems such as Scleroderma (a skin disease). The Proetz procedure has been used by ear, nose and throat surgeons for years to clean out the sinuses during surgery.

Nasal rinsing (*lavage*) devices have included gravity flow vessels, pressure bottles, IV bags, squirts, flushers, syringes, electrical machines, squeeze bottles and turkey basters, among others. Some people mistakenly include misters, sprays and humidifiers among nasal irrigation devices but let's make this perfectly clear: they are not. One is a flowing cleansing flush; the other is a mild misting or spray.

Interest in the idea of nasal cleansing grew slowly in the mid to late 1990's. Since the new millennium, this interest has exploded, powered by the surge in prevention-focused medicine, alternative therapies, and an overall integrative approach to health. Well-known doctors have promoted the practice of nasal washing. Although antihistamines, decongestants, steroids and antibiotics are commonly prescribed, doctors have added the adjunctive treatment of nasal irrigation for allergy sufferers, post-operative sinus surgery patients and for those who suffer from chronic sinusitis. I have advocated nasal washing for more than two decades, but only recently has it been formally recommended as a mainstream preventative approach.

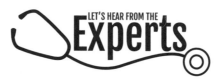

I have asked P. Leszek Vincent, Ph.D., for his perspective on the history and the origins of nasal washing. Dr. Vincent is a research professor who has studied traditional remedies through the ages and has considerable expertise in the history and use of medicinal plants. He has studied in South Africa, the United Kingdom and the United States and has written several publications on medicinal plants.

Nose Washing Through the Ages

Nasal washing, or nasal irrigation, is an ancient Ayurvedic technique known as Jala neti, which literally means "nasal cleansing" in Sanskrit (a classical language of South Asia). With origins based in the yoga tradition, nasal washing has been used throughout India and South East Asia. Although not commonly practiced by Western cultures, these Eastern cultures have performed Jala neti as routinely as brushing one's teeth for centuries. Yogic breathing practices, known as pranayama, are enhanced by the practice of Jala neti since many of them involve deep breathing through the nostrils, and clear nasal passages permit deeper, more relaxed breathing.

Traditionally a neti pot, a vessel shaped like an Aladdin's lamp or teapot, has been used to flow salt water into one nostril, and out the other nostril. In addition to using the neti pot, ancient yogis experienced success by snorting salt water in a rhythmic fashion as part of their daily rituals.

In the West, doctors have known the benefits of nasal washing for more than a century. The first mention of nasal irrigation in western medical literature is in an article published in 1902 in the British medical journal The Lancet. This article also mentions the inclusion of "a pinch of sodium bicarbonate" to the warm saline solution as the bicarbonate can improve the quality of the cleansing action of the nasal wash solution. Interestingly this article also mentions the value of using boiled seawater as a nasal wash solution. Coastal cultures around the world provide much anecdotal information about the value of swimming in the sea or sniffing sea water up into the nose when suffering from a cold or other nasal congestion problem. Note that the salt content of seawater is approximately 3.5% while that of a hypertonic saline solution, typically used in current nasal washing practice, ranges from 3 to 5%. Recent medical research has demonstrated that nasal irrigation using a hypertonic saline solution promotes the body's cleaning of the mucous membranes in our noses, via stimulating the cleaning action of the minute hairs that are found on the surface of the mucous membranes in our nasal passages (mucociliary clearance). It is interesting that the human practice of nasal washing, while having ancient roots, is founded upon sound medical and scientific principles.

P. Leszek Vincent, PhD, FLS
Research Assistant Professor
Division of Plant Sciences
University of Missouri

The Evolution of

Device	Description	Flow	Date
	Neti	Gravity	> three millennium
	Dr Sage's Nasal Douche	Gravity	1890s
	Glass Bottle with air port	Gravity	1902
	Upright Vessel	Gravity	1915
	Double Portal	Gravity	1917
	Benjamin Nasal Douche	Gravity	1930's

Medical Nasal Devices

Device	Description	Flow	Date
	Upright Bottle	Gravity	1990's
	Pulsating Mechanical Irrigation	Forced pressure	~ 2000
	Squeeze Bottle with Billow	Positive pressure, against gravity	~ 2004
	Squeeze Bottle with Straw	Positive pressure, against gravity	2001
	Dr Hana's Nasopure Bottle	Gravity & positive pressure	2004

Chapter 5

The Ins and Outs of Nasal Washing — Taking Care of Your Great Defender

 Nasal washing is easily learned and just like most skills, becomes easier with practice. It is not difficult to master, and when performed correctly, it is a refreshing and soothing experience. It is analogous to brushing your teeth, flossing, or learning to use contact lenses.

Let's be clear here: nasal "irrigation" systems ARE NOT: sprayers, sniffing water, misters, nebulizers, gels, humidifiers, bulb syringes (mold grows easily inside these) or other devices that spray or moisturize only. Nor can nasal washing be accomplished by "snorting" water into the nose.

Why Wash Daily?

✓ Daily practice of washing improves both nasal and sinus health.

✓ Washes out thick and sticky mucus.

✓ Thins thick and sticky secretions.

✓ Reduces nasal congestion.

✓ Improves air flow.

✓ Improves filter efficiency.

✓ Allows the sinus cavities to drain freely.

✓ Removes allergens, irritants, bacteria, viruses and contaminants.

✓ Helps reduce upper respiratory infections like the common cold.

✓ May reduce dependency on medications (antibiotics, antihistamines, nasal steroids, decongestants, asthma medications).

✓ Relieves nasal dryness.

✓ Can improve sense of smell.

- ✓ Can improve sense of taste.
- ✓ Helps to treat sinusitis and rhinitis.
- ✓ Reduces allergic rhinitis symptoms.
- ✓ Reduces coughing and other symptoms of post-nasal drip.
- ✓ May reduce snoring.
- ✓ May reduce nose bleeds.
- ✓ Helps heal raw or irritated nasal membranes.
- ✓ Clears airways affected by nose woes associated with pregnancy and aging.
- ✓ Helps clear excessive mucus caused by medical conditions such as Cystic Fibrosis.
- ✓ Cleanses the nasal tissues stressed by radiation therapy to the head and sinus area.
- ✓ Removes pollutants from the upper airway to allow deeper, more relaxed breathing.
- ✓ Feels soothing and refreshing; a *shower for the nose.*
- ✓ It's easy, inexpensive, and makes sense.

Who Should Wash?

 Now, who should wash their nose? Well, consider this: who should brush their teeth? People with teeth, right? The simple answer is that just about anyone who has a nose should wash their nose, and I'm being serious. Beyond this broad group, people who have particular concerns will appreciate dramatic benefits from daily nose washing. I'm talking about people who have:

- ✓ Sinus issues
- ✓ Nose issues
- ✓ Throat issues
- ✓ Asthma
- ✓ Post nasal drip (PND)
- ✓ Allergies
- ✓ Ear infections

- ✓ Sinus surgery/nasal surgery
- ✓ Irritating or non-allergic rhinitis (chemical or other airborne irritant to the nose)
- ✓ Seasoned noses
- ✓ Cystic Fibrosis (CF)
- ✓ Lack of or decreased sense of smell or taste
- ✓ Bad breath (from excessive infected mucus)
- ✓ Snoring issues
- ✓ Pregnancy rhinitis
- ✓ CPAP users, for sleep apnea

...as well as

- ✓ Athletes, including but not limited to runners, football players, baseball players, soccer players, golfers, scuba divers, horseback riders
- ✓ Farmers and gardeners
- ✓ Travelers
- ✓ Workers in environments with poor or potentially harmful air quality such as firefighters, construction workers, painters, military personnel
- ✓ People who live in polluted cities
- ✓ Those interested in using fewer drugs and saving money
- ✓ Anyone interested in prevention: cleaning their personal filter
- ✓ Anyone who speaks frequently or sings for a living

...and that's just a partial list.

Dr. Hana's
CLINICAL PEARLS

Nasal Issues? Wash The Tissues!

Who Should NOT Wash?

✓ Those who are unable to stand alone and brush their teeth.

✓ Anyone who can't follow instructions.

✓ Those who have had recent trauma or surgery to the head or neck.

✓ Anyone with a physician who says, "No nasal washing for you!"

✓ Anyone who is being forced to use a nasal wash against their will.

When to Wash?

✓ Allergy season.

✓ Cold and flu season for prevention.

✓ At the first sign of nasal congestion.

✓ Immediately after exposure to irritants and pollutants.

✓ If infected in the ears, sinus, nose or throat.

✓ During asthma flare-ups.

✓ When your sense of smell and/or taste is impaired.

✓ Before use of nasal steroids or other nasal medications.

✓ Before using CPAP machines for sleep apnea.

✓ Every day as part of general hygiene practice.

How Frequently to Wash?

Dr. Hana's
CLINICAL ⬤ PEARLS

Frequency of washing depends on your need,
your goals, and your motivation.

For Prevention:
Wash once per day *and* after exposure to irritants.

For Mild to Moderate Congestion or Discharge:
Wash twice per day.

For Moderate to Severe Congestion, Discharge or Infection:
Wash up to four times per day.

Cleaner! Clearer!

66 *I could immediately tell a difference in my nose, feeling just clearer to breathe after one use! I thought my whole family needed to try this.* 99

Paul K, Wichita, Kansas

Gift of Clear Air

66 *Both my mother and dad love nose washing. They got theirs for Christmas and Mom says it is the best thing ever invented.* 99

Michelle B., Homecare Specialist, North Carolina

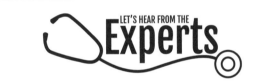

LET'S HEAR FROM THE
Experts

The frequency of nasal washing with buffered hypertonic nasal saline irrigation is related to the severity of the disease. Patients with mild disease can irrigate only as needed for comfort. Patients with severe disease should irrigate three to four times each day or even more. The duration of nasal washings in days or weeks or months also depends on the severity of the disease and contributing factors such as allergies, colds, frequency of being around smokers, etc.

David S. Parsons, MD, FAAP, FACS, Clinical Professor,
Universities of North and South Carolina, Pediatric Otolaryngology,
Charlotte Eye, Ear, Nose, and Throat Associates

What to Wash With

There are two qualities in a nasal wash solution that make an enormous difference: salt concentration and acidity. But first, the water you use should be previously boiled, purified, distilled or otherwise sterilized. I am not personally concerned about my own tap water, and I use tap water for myself, but officially I recommend sterilized water for all nasal wash solutions.

Mucous membranes and the mucus produced in the nose are both naturally salty; an effective wash will take that saltiness into account. In addition, if the solution washing over the membranes is too acidic it will be irritating rather than soothing to the membranes. These factors are quite important, so we are going to take some time to explore both of them.

Solutions and Salt Facts You Should Know

Before we discuss salt concentrations, we need to review some basic physiology. The body has membranes that allow water to cross from one side to the other and as a result, we experience shrinking and swelling of those membranes. The diffusion or natural movement of water across a membrane is called *osmosis*.

When a permeable membrane like we have in our nose is washed with salty solution, the high salt content draws the excess liquid from the less salty side into the more salty side, in an attempt to equalize the concentration of salt on each side. Water moves through osmosis towards the highest salt content, coming out of the mucous membranes and, in effect, shrinking those membranes down.

When salt is concentrated inside or outside the cell membranes, it will draw the water in its direction. Here's a good example of this phenomenon: have you ever made coleslaw out of cabbage? Cabbage salad is best when crispy, not soggy. My mother knew that the way to make good coleslaw was to shred the cabbage and then cover it with liberal amounts of salt. When she returned a few minutes later to rinse the salted and shredded cabbage she knew that the bowl would be full of water. This water was the fluid extracted from the cabbage, leaving it crunchy and perfect for a salad.

Salt absorbs, it draws, it drinks, it extracts, and it sucks the water from its surroundings. In our nose there is evidence that salty solutions pull liquid out of swollen tissue, thus unplugging the sinus and inner ear openings, resulting in natural draining of mucus. Salty solutions also transform thick sticky mucus into a thinner consistency making drainage easier.

Saline is a generic term referring to a mixture of salt and water. But this term does not reflect how many salt particles are in a given volume of water, i.e. the strength of the saline. The strength of saline is referred to as *tonicity*. Saline can be hypertonic, isotonic or hypotonic.

The body is the standard against which we gauge other salt mixtures; the salt concentration in the body is 0.9%. If a solution is identical to the salt concentration in the body, it is referred to as *isotonic*. If there is more salt as compared to the body, the solution is *hypertonic* and if there is less salt than the body it is *hypotonic*. The differences are amazing and worth understanding in detail.

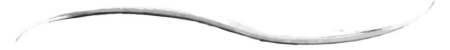

Dr. Hana's
CLINICAL ⬤ PEARLS

Water follows salt;
use salty water when you want the most effective wash.

Hypertonic Nasal Wash Solution

Hypertonic means the salt solution is saltier than the body's natural state.

Scientific studies have shown that hypertonic nasal wash solution has numerous benefits:

- ✓ Shrinks membranes with osmosis by pulling fluid out of swollen tissues.
- ✓ Improves mucus flow.
- ✓ Thins thick sticky secretions.
- ✓ Improves the filtering efficiency of the nose.
- ✓ Washes out irritants that cause allergies.
- ✓ Is as safe as ocean water.
- ✓ Can improve both sense of smell and bad breath.
- ✓ Reduces the need for some medications when used on a regular basis.
- ✓ Reduces the frequency of the common cold if used regularly.

We also know that a high salt concentration (hypertonic) inhibits and kills viruses and bacteria. Washing the nasal cavities with a salty solution after exposure to a cold, or when fighting an infection, has been shown to reduce the number of infectious particles. A hypertonic solution impedes infectious particles attempting to invade mucous membranes. It also reduces viral multiplication.

Sometimes washing with a hypertonic solution can be irritating to the nasal mucosa. I believe this experience can be related to several factors which include age, hormone levels, medication effects, and nasal history. This irritation is almost always temporary and causes no damage to the mucous membranes.

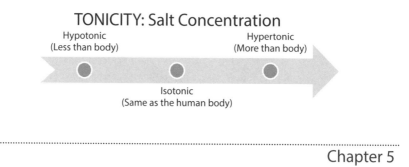

TONICITY: Salt Concentration

Hypotonic
(Less than body)

Hypertonic
(More than body)

Isotonic
(Same as the human body)

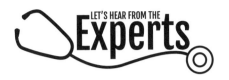

Isotonic Nasal Wash Solution

Isotonic means the concentration of salt is equal on both sides of a membrane. When the body's salt concentration is the same as the washing solution, the solution will not have any effect on the overall amount of water on either side of the mucous membrane. Thus, this will not shrink swollen membranes. An isotonic concentration of salt solution can physically remove some irritants, but will not inhibit infections or thin the secretions. Some prefer the isotonic solution; it is a milder mix and feels comfortable when used daily but does not have as many benefits as hypertonic saline. Many people like to begin nasal washing with an isotonic solution, and advance to hypertonic as tolerated.

Benefits of Isotonic Solution

- ✓ Easily tolerated.
- ✓ Makes an excellent maintenance nose wash.

Comparison of Hypertonic vs. Isotonic

	Hypertonic 3.0% Salinity	Isotonic 0.9% Salinity
Mucus	Transforms Jelly-like and sticky mucus to thin and watery substance	No change
Membranes	Shrinks swelling of nasal membranes	No change
Debris	Releases and removes debris from membranes and cilia	Removes from membranes
Cilia	Improves transit time by 17%	No change
Allergens	80% of inflammatory mediators washed away	Unclear
Bacteria and Virus	Inhibits growth and invasion into mucosal lining	No effect
Biofilm*	Helps removes film	No effect
Medication	Decreased	Some decrease

* See pg 80 (Biofilms)

Hypotonic Nasal Wash Solution

Hypotonic means the salt concentration in the solution contains less salt than the body. Regular tap water is hypotonic. Remember *osmosis*? When the solution is less salty than the membranes, the fluid will move to the saltier side - in this case, to the inside of the membrane. Washing with a hypotonic solution can actually cause increased swelling of the nasal and sinus membranes. You may have noticed this effect if you have ever tried to wash your nose with plain water instead of a salty solution. Washing with hypotonic solution is *not* and *never has* been recommended.

Buffering, pH and Acidity

Okay, back to some basic chemistry. Hang in here - it's pretty simple and well worth understanding.

The pH level is a number that indicates levels of alkalinity and acidity. The abbreviation pH means "power of hydrogen," which is a chemist's way of looking at relative acidity. In pH language, 7 is neutral; lower than that is acidic and higher than that is alkaline. You may have seen the "pH scale" on a test strip for your swimming pool or spa. The lower the pH, the more acidic your pool water is. Higher pH means the water is alkaline. The nasal membranes have a pH of about 5.3-7.0, on the acid side of neutral. Typical tap water has a pH of about 6, also on the acidic side of the scale.

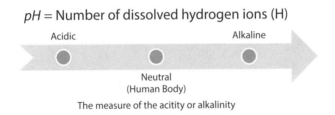

pH = Number of dissolved hydrogen ions (H)

Acidic

Alkaline

Neutral
(Human Body)

The measure of the acitity or alkalinity

Now, what does *buffer* mean? A *buffer* is a chemical that keeps something where it should be. It prevents adverse swings. It shields, cushions and protects. And in the case of nose washing solutions, buffering adjusts and sets the pH for the most comfortable and effective washing solution. If the solution is alkaline, with a higher pH, the high salt content is easily tolerated by the mucous membranes. If one washes with a very salty solution but one devoid of buffering, it will sting.

Bicarbonate raises the pH of water (~ 6) to a more alkaline level (7.5-8.5) which is definitely beneficial. Bicarbonate helps soothe irritated membranes, and we are more likely to keep using a solution that feels good. Studies have shown that buffering also increases the efficiency of ciliary clearance and augments healing.

Sometimes people who are congested and irritated by inflammation find that even neutral salt may sting the raw nasal passages a bit. We do know that the saline wash actually augments healing and that this uncomfortable sensation is very temporary. Often the second or third washing will feel comfortable. Therefore, I suggest always beginning with an isotonic solution and advancing to hypertonic as tolerated. Most people can advance within three days, easily tolerating and enjoying the sensation of a cleaner nose.

Benefits of Buffered Solutions

- Higher pH with sodium bicarbonate improves mucus flow.
- Augments healing of tissues.
- Soothes membranes.
- Increases tolerance to very salty solutions.
- Dramatically increases amounts of "inflammatory mediators" (allergens) removed during nasal washing.

Dr. Talbot and Dr. Parsons, two eminent ear, nose and throat specialists, have incorporated buffered hypertonic saline nasal irrigation into the care of their patients with acute and chronic sinusitis. They strongly recommend it for those having undergone sinus surgery. In their 1997 study, the ciliary function in various saline environments was evaluated and they concluded the following: "The outcome showed buffered hypertonic saline nasal irrigation to improve mucociliary transit times, while buffered normal saline had no such effect. Buffered hypertonic saline nasal irrigation is an important addition to the care of sinus disease".

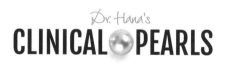

Dr. Hana's

CLINICAL PEARLS

Hypertonic buffered wash is the most effective.

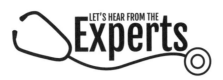

David S Parsons, MD specializes in adults and children with difficult sinus problems, and in pediatric ear, nose, and throat care. He wrote and edited one of the best-selling books in the world on sinus care, and created three internationally distributed CD-ROMs describing comprehensive sinus care, emphasizing the Minimally Invasive Surgical Technique, which he helped develop.

For time longer than we know (at least three millennia), salt water has been used for nasal irrigation. When the amount of salt in a specific volume of water is the same as what is in your blood, we call it "saline." When the nose is washed with saline, we call this a "balanced solution" because the amount of salt on either side of your nasal membrane is the same. But we questioned how a balanced solution can reduce nasal swelling. We performed tests comparing saline to "hypertonic saline," or an unbalanced solution with more salt than is in your blood.

Our findings were unexpected. Patients felt the high salt concentration was much better, but clearly stated they would not use it, because it burned the inside of their nose. Therefore, we buffered it with bicarbonate. Patients, including young children, informed us that we now offered the best solution they had ever used.

We then performed a number of studies to measure objectively the true benefits of Buffered Hypertonic Nasal Saline Irrigation. Every study done revealed that this solution was superior to either normal saline, water, or un-buffered hypertonic saline. Finally, we tested a variety of strengths for the optimal solution and clearly showed that three times the amount of salt than is in your blood is best. The amount of bicarbonate was enough to raise the pH one unit (from about 6.4 to 7.4) thus creating an alkaline solution.

Further studies by an independent lab revealed that the frequency of the beating of little cilia (hair-like structures on each cell surface) increased ten to twelve times/minute resulting in much better clearance of secretions from both the nose and the sinuses. This was most unexpected. We were only trying to keep the nose from burning but the side benefits of the bicarbonate were very impressive.

Over the years, we have received letters and emails from all over the world from happy users of this product. The patients and parents report a decreased need for emergency room visits, fewer antibiotics, few x-rays, less discomfort and a healthier state of being.

Our interest in this product was purely from a standpoint of trying to find the best care for our patients. None of our research team ever received a penny from any of the products available using this recipe. We have no financial interest in any company that produces this product. But we know that it works better than any other solution available... and so do our patients.

David S. Parsons, MD, FAAP, FACS Clinical Professor,
Universities of North and South Carolina,
Pediatric Otolaryngology, Charlotte Eye, Ear,
Nose, and Throat Associates

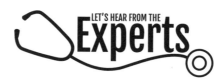

Advantages of Hypertonic Solution

Nasal washing inflamed and swollen sinuses is most effective when solutions contain high salt concentrations. Concentrated salt solutions are known to shrink swollen tissues to enhance drainage and to stop bacterial putrification (salt preserving as in salt pork). Gargling with salty water speeds a sore throat to recover. Many bacteria including Staph Aureus contain a higher salt concentration than our blood. Antibiotics that work to weaken bacterial cell walls allow water to move osmotically into bacteria to make them swell up and burst. High salt may also weaken ionic bonds by which bacteria adhere to epithelial cells.

Our own white blood cells use hydrogen peroxide to destroy many types of dangerous bacteria such as Staphylococcus aureus (SA) and methicillin resistant SA (MRSA). For MRSA skin infections, salty peroxide solutions are being recommended. Likewise, nasal washing devices can deliver diluted

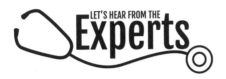

LET'S HEAR FROM THE Experts

Benjamin D. Francisco, PhD and nurse practitioner, specializes in pediatric allergy, asthma and Cystic Fibrosis in a large teaching hospital. His experience includes a keen interest in prevention and education. Dr. Francisco has become a leader in this field and lectures extensively to doctors, nurses and respiratory therapists.

Use of hypertonic nasal rinses has reduced the need for more invasive and risky treatments in our clinical practice. When the nose is in good condition it is protective against a range of other problems, including worsening asthma, shortness of breath with exertion related to nasal obstruction, and the development of bacterial infections in the sinuses.

Those who master good technique have great results and do not feel like rinsing the nose is a problem. On the other hand, those who do not master good technique often feel that this is a terrible thing to have to do. In my clinical practice I have parents with children as young as three years of age that tell me their child brings their rinse bottle to their mother saying that they want to rinse their nose. Then we have, of course, teens that run screaming when they see the rinse bottle.

I consider it important to introduce the technique in a way that is acceptable, giving people a clear mental image of what they are doing. The method that I currently use emphasizes that when you rinse your nose the most important thing is to first establish an air stream out of the free nostril before you squeeze the bottle and push a column of water into the other nostril. Failure to provide a ready outlet for the incoming stream of salt water can cause unpleasant effects including gagging and possible ear pain, because increased pressure in the throat is transmitted to the Eustachian tube and middle ear.

Very young children present a special challenge to parents. However, if a child can blow their nose, I think they can easily adapt to the nasal rinsing technique described above. I use this method in clinic. Starting with air only I demonstrate the technique with young children and youths, asking that they lean forward and blow air slowly out of one nostril while I puff a little air from the irrigation bottle into the other nostril. We switch sides and repeat the procedure. I explain that practicing with air will make it easier to master the real thing at home with salt water.

It is also helpful to understand that inside each nostril are three nasal turbinates. If the first turbinate is enlarged, then nasal steroids or nasal antihistamine sprays will not enter the upper nasal passages effectively. Instead, medication will strike the first turbinate and then flow back out, failing to have any impact on the other two turbinates or the lining of the upper nasal passages. This is confirmed by anecdotal reports by families and children in my practice when they say, "My medicine is not going in. It just streams back out of my nose even if I try to inhale or sniff it into the back of my nose." Rinsing the nose with hypertonic salt water before using the spray decongests and shrinks the turbinates, thus improving delivery of nasal medications.

I think it's also important to explain that use of hypertonic saline is like swimming in the ocean and having some salt water washing in and out of the nostrils. I compare rinsing the nose with salt water to swimming in the ocean - except we are bringing the ocean to you in a small bottle.

Salt-water rinses also wash away secretions and debris (pollen, dust and other stuff in the air we breathe) that are contributing to nasal congestion. This is a common problem for school age children who play outdoors after school during mold and pollen season. When they come indoors, if the nose is doing its job, there is a considerable amount of allergen particles (spores or pollen) in the nose. If these are rinsed out it is likely that this will lessen the allergic response. Walking around with this stuff in your nose for hours cannot be a good thing.

A final effect, and in my mind the most important benefit of salt water rinses, is stimulation of the natural sweepers that line the sinus passages. This effect results in improved mucociliary clearance, the natural system for washing the sinuses clear by moving secretions out of the nasal airways.

As an adjunct to treating sinus infections, nasal rinses with hypertonic salt water are valuable. People recover more quickly and are more likely to have a complete cure, even when antibiotics are also indicated. Future sinus infections might be averted and the need for antibiotics avoided if the person is comfortable using salt water rinses to aid body defenses in the future.

I am so convinced of the benefit of hypertonic salt-water rinses that I provide starter kits at no cost to families (hundreds of kits over the course of the last four years). I tell families that if they begin to rinse the nose for a period of a week or so when nasal congestion first occurs, there is a strong possibility that antibiotics may not be needed next time. I generally recommend a one-week period of daily nasal rinsing once or twice a day, preferably twice. I am more inclined to recommend rinsing the nose twice a day if the nasal symptoms are more severe or if they are not improving with once daily rinsing. Some people ask if they can rinse more often and the answer is yes.

I hope more will acquire this skill and use nasal rinsing as a routine part of their hygiene and wellness.

Benjamin D. Francisco, PhD, PNP, AE-C
Research Assistant Professor of Child Health Pulmonary Medicine
and AllergyUniversity of Missouri Health Care

Additives for Your Nose Wash Solution?

I am often asked if you should add anything to your salt solution to make nasal washing more effective. Well, what's your preference? Some like it mild and some like it stronger. Salt solutions come in many variations and occasionally people like to add additional ingredients to their wash at home. Some of these ingredients have been proven by adequate research to be helpful. Others may not have been scientifically proven to be helpful but on the other hand, appear to do no harm. Then there are a few that should be avoided.

Before you start considering additives in your wash solution, most important to remember is Environmental Control. Doing what you can, both inside and outside your home and workplace, is the first step to protecting your nose. Decrease the toxic load your filter has to deal with so you don't even get to that tipping point where symptoms overwhelm you. Air filters for the air you breathe, bed linens washed in hot water to destroy dust mites, and avoidance of known allergens can all make a difference if allergies are your main culprit. Then, washing your nose to remove the toxins you can't avoid will be most effective.

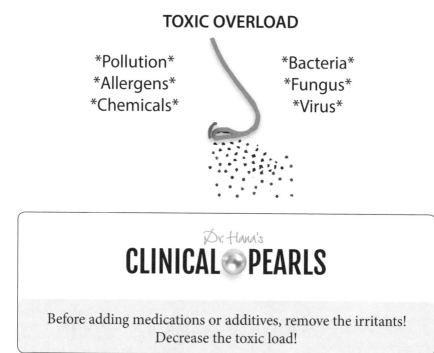

TOXIC OVERLOAD

Pollution
Allergens
Chemicals

Bacteria
Fungus
Virus

Dr. Hana's
CLINICAL PEARLS

Before adding medications or additives, remove the irritants!
Decrease the toxic load!

The information in this chapter should not be considered an endorsement for any specific product. It includes information both old and new, with much of it considered folklore, passed down but not scientifically proven. Common sense leads me to believe that some of the essential oils may be harmful if accidentally inhaled and some of the herbal remedies may indeed trigger allergies in susceptible individuals. I suggest you do your own investigation, consider the risks and benefits of each additive, ask your medical provider, or if uncertain, play it safe and use a prepared solution proven to do no harm.

Use these additives with caution after you are well informed about their use.

Proven Helpful in Scientific Studies

Xylitol

Xylitol is a sugar alcohol found in many fruits and vegetables, also produced in small amounts by the human body. It is as sweet as glucose sugar and manufactured from birch trees in Finland, cane bagasse, and corncobs.

Bacteria and yeasts can metabolize regular glucose sugar but they cannot metabolize xylitol. The structure of xylitol prevents it.

If xylitol is on the lining of the mucous membranes it prevents bacteria from sticking to the inside of your nose and throat. In 2004, this fact was proved in a study that exposed rabbits to nasal bacteria in both nostrils. One nostril was washed with plain saline solution and the other washed with saline that also had xylitol in it. The xylitol/saline solution clearly protected the rabbits from getting a bacterial infection. This indicates that xylitol may have a role in *preventing* infections, but we do not yet know if it can *treat* a sinus infection.

There is a suggestion by some that chewing xylitol gum may help prevent ear infections. Two possible mechanisms may account for this. The act of chewing helps open and close the Eustachian tubes, encouraging ventilation. In addition, as shown in the previously mentioned study, xylitol helps prevent the growth of bacteria in the Eustachian tubes.

Too much xylitol can become toxic. It acts as a laxative and can actually cause low blood sugar. Too much of anything is never good.

Baby Shampoo and Biofilms

Once bacteria sets up shop in the nose, they will sometimes go further and create a community of bacteria combined with the body's own white blood cells (the cells that fight infection). This community is called a *biofilm* - a protective slimy matrix often stuck to the mucous membranes like plaque on teeth or the slippery slime on river stones. Biofilms allow bacteria to easily multiply and to recruit other bacteria to join them. *Staphylococcus aureus* and *Pseudomonas aeruginosa*, two common culprits in sinus infections, are especially good at creating biofilms.

Bacteria in a biofilm require 1000 times the concentration of antibiotics than those not in a biofilm. Biofilms also make bacteria resistant to our own immune system. This situation leads to chronic sinusitis. But the right kind of nasal wash can win the battle against biofilms!

To rid the sinus and nose of chronic infection, the biofilm must be broken and recent studies have shown that a simple surfactant can do just that. Surfactants contain both water-soluble and water-insoluble components and this helps them break chemical bonds that hold biofilms together. The best news?

A common and easily obtainable surfactant is baby shampoo free of perfume and additives. Baby shampoo is well tolerated and safe to use as a surfactant additive to your wash. Just a few drops added to a saline nose wash can break up biofilms, allowing antibiotics and the immune system to do their job. This can be used occasionally for prevention. For those suffering from chronic infections, daily use of one or two drops of surfactant in an eight ounce nasal wash solution can prevent biofilms from forming in the first place.

Antibiotics/Antifungal Agents

Pharmacists and doctors may recommend the addition of antibiotics to nasal wash solutions, delivering the medication directly to the infected areas. Delivery right to the infected area offers some benefits. For example, this approach reduces the body's total exposure to the antibiotics. Additionally, direct washing with antibiotics eliminates the destruction of normal intestinal balance. Finally, topical use in a nasal wash instead of systemic use with pills may reduce the incidence of allergic reactions to antibiotics.

Used, Supported By Traditional Use, But Lacking In Scientific Evidence

Hydrogen peroxide (H2O2) can be used to rinse nasal cavities. It is a simple molecule - just water with one extra highly reactive oxygen atom. When hydrogen peroxide enters a bacterial cell, this highly reactive oxygen molecule wreaks havoc, destabilizing the cell to the point of destruction. This destroys bacterial cells because bacteria lack catalase, a chemical which breaks down hydrogen peroxide into simple water and oxygen. Humans are not harmed because our cells have a chemical called catalase, which easily breaks down hydrogen peroxide into simple water and oxygen.

Dilute solutions of 3% hydrogen peroxide are very inexpensive and available at any drug store. Although many individuals swear it works, there is no scientific support for the effectiveness of a hydrogen peroxide wash. I would not suggest this for children or those with sensitive nasal passages.

Manuka honey is made by bees from Manuka flowers in New Zealand and has some unique properties that make it attractive for use in nasal wash solutions. It is a powerful anti-inflammatory, helps cut through biofilms, and has wound healing properties.

Manuka honey has more than one quality that allows it to act as a natural antibiotic. It draws water out of bacteria, drying them out so they cannot survive. Honey is also acidic and the lower pH prevents further bacterial growth. And when the sugar in honey metabolizes, it produces hydrogen peroxide - an excellent antiseptic.

If you add a tablespoon of mildly warmed Manuka honey to an eight ounce bottle of hypertonic wash solution it can be effective when needed to prevent chronic sinusitis. But you don't want to use Manuka honey in your nasal wash every single day; your cilia won't like it. Just like prescription antibiotics and other medications, honey should only be used when needed. And never overheat honey - it kills some of the healing properties.

Berberine botanicals are plant alkaloids that have been used for centuries in Ayurvedic and Chinese medicine. They are found in the roots and stem bark of many healing plants, including Goldenseal (Hydrastis canadensis), Oregon grape (Berberis aquifolium), Barberry (Berberis vulgaris) and Tree turmeric (Berberis aristata). Berberine extracts and decoctions have been shown to have excellent antimicrobial properties against bacteria, viruses and fungi. Berberine botanicals also act as anti-inflammatory agents.

Adding berberine extracts to your nasal wash solution may increase the beneficial effects and although there are no studies to prove this, it does have many years of common usage to support its healing effects.

Quercetin is a chemical found naturally in wine and many fruits and vegetables. We know it works well as an anti-inflammatory, and it has some anti-viral properties.

The cells that release histamines when we have allergic reactions are called *mast cells*. Quercetin may work to stabilize these mast cells to help block the release of histamine that causes inflammation. Added to nasal wash solutions, it could help prevent seasonal allergic reactions.

Lab tests on quercetin are promising, but no reliable research has been done to see how well it might work for people. Adding a little to a hypertonic saline wash solution may help prevent allergic reactions.

Grapefruit seed extract is made from the pulp of the seeds of grapefruits, and reportedly has strong antibacterial, antifungal and anti-candida properties. There appears to be no harm in adding this to your hypertonic nasal wash solution, and it may help prevent or heal a sinus infection. Grapefruit seed extract is one of my personal favorites.

Aromatherapy and essential oils can be quite powerful and they should be respected for their potential to both heal and harm. Some suggest very small amounts may be helpful if included in a nasal wash solution, but anyone using them should pay special attention to all safety precautions before use. Tea Tree Oil probably has antibacterial and antifungal properties. Eucalyptus Oil may reduce inflammation if you add a couple of drops to each bottle of hypertonic saline solution.

Essential oils: points to remember

- ✓ Use with caution around children.
- ✓ Remember, oils are flammable.
- ✓ Monitor for reactions to aromatic oils. When using for the first time, use only a single drop to test for sensitivity.
- ✓ Review all safety instructions.
- ✓ Learn about and understand the properties of each essential oil prior to use.

Caution!

Colloidal silver is a liquid suspension of submicroscopic particles of silver. It is known that silver has antibacterial properties but toxicity is a significant and serious concern. The usefulness of silver for nasal irrigation is highly controversial. Colloidal silver was used as a mainstream antibiotic prior to the 1930s and it has a long history as a disinfectant for hospitals, but this use was discontinued decades ago due to significant side effects. Long-term use of silver preparations can lead to irreversible silver toxicity (*argyria* where the skin turns ashen-gray with silver salt deposits in the skin, eyes and internal organs).

Silver nitrate was applied throughout the 20th century to newborns' eyes to prevent infection but that usage was discontinued many years ago. Topical silver sulfadiazine creams have been used in burn centers for many years and continue to be used effectively today.

Many patients continue to insist that silver is a helpful additive, but when I weigh the risks and benefits, and when I consider the availability of other effective but less worrisome additives, I must advise that silver not be used in nasal wash solutions unless under the close supervision of a knowledgeable provider.

Finally, to summarize: various nasal rinse combinations have been studied, including isotonic and hypertonic saline, with and without buffering, with additives that include those discussed above. Consistently, hypertonic buffered saline solution has proven to be effective for congestion from any source. Isotonic buffered saline works well for overall daily washing.

Nose Wash Style — So Many Choices! How to Choose?

 Nasal irrigation can be carried out through a variety of methods. Some people think nose washing is the same as sniffing salt water from a cupped hand; some think it is the same as using an infant's suction bulb. But these methods are not really irrigation, they are simply moisturization. Many more options are available today for those who are serious about daily washing. There are three general major types of actual nasal irrigation:

✓ Gravity based systems, like the neti, allow the flow of fluid to drain into and out of the nasal and sinus cavities. There is no positive pressure. This comes with the disadvantage of less control of the fluid flow and therefore, difficulty in flushing when congested.

✓ Positive-pressure irrigation means that the solution is propelled into the nose. This is achieved by a syringe type device, a squeeze bottle device that propels the solution against gravity, or a squeeze bottle device that propels along with gravity. Some systems offer the user control of flow pressure.

✓ A motorized device designed specifically for irrigation uses both positive-pressure and pulsatile irrigation. This is very effective but can be expensive, and machines tend to be neither child friendly nor travel ready.

The Importance of Head Position

 Both the wash system as well as the head and neck's position determine the direction of flushing. Some systems encourage flow along the nasal floor, in the same path as the air we breathe, while others flush upward into the sinus cavities. In addition, if you have to bend or twist your neck to create a flow, it can cause neck pain, dizziness or a lack of control. Children and older adults are among those most susceptible to problems with head positioning.

I have to confess, I'm not a natural swimmer nor do I enjoy the feeling of jumping into water and flooding my head and sinuses. Ouch! How can I get my two-year-old patients to wash regularly? It has to feel good.

I always instruct my patients to wash, as I personally prefer, with a straight neck, no bending or twisting of the neck *(neutral neck)* and head in line with the rest of the spine. When the solution flow follows the natural direction of airflow, along the nasal floor, the feeling is comfortable, with no sensation of choking or drowning. This flushing, where positive pressure is constant, sets up a negative pressure area outside of the sinus openings resulting in an evacuation of the sinus cavity. This encourages mucus to drain outward. No fluid enters into the sinus cavity. (See Chapter 6)

In systems that flush upward, the solution can enter the sinus cavities. This may result in a feeling of increased head pressure. Many experts believe this upward direction of flow washes the dirt, along with solution, into the sinus cavity. Hopefully, these irritating particles will exit with the mucus when the solution drains.

The position of the head during nose washing is determined by the type of irrigation system being used. You can see a clear comparison of systems and necessary head positions in the figures on the next page.

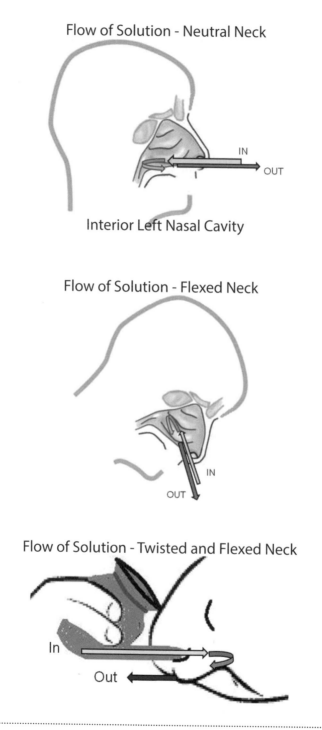

Flow of Solution - Neutral Neck

IN

OUT

Interior Left Nasal Cavity

Flow of Solution - Flexed Neck

IN

OUT

Flow of Solution - Twisted and Flexed Neck

In

Out

Consider the Volume

 Washing can be accomplished by using small amounts of water or larger irrigation flows. Imagine a dirty, congested nose. You can spray some water onto the tissues, and this may add a few droplets of moisture but it will not cleanse like a full flush with continuously flowing water.

When you are first learning to wash, use a small squirt through each nostril, just enough to have a bit of solution exit the opposite side. Often as little as one ounce per side is adequate. If you already are an experienced nose washer, or congested, or exposed to infection or pollution, two to three ounces can be used. If you suspect or have been diagnosed with an infection of the nose, sinuses, ears or asthma flare up, you may find a full four ounces is needed. Some prefer smaller volumes while others enjoy the feeling of a continuous washing. Follow your comfort instincts and never force any fluid; it should go in easily. As you gain confidence, let comfort be your guide.

Technique and Style

 First-time washers should always begin with a small amount of warm washing solution and increase as your personal preference directs. Over the sink or in the shower is the best place to learn how to wash. A mirror can help guide you in regards to the device and head position.

If your bottle or other device has a tip that allows a complete seal against your nostril you will have a more thorough and controlled washing experience. When you are able to create a good seal, the solution is encouraged to flow out the other side of the nose, creating the most effective wash. Use your mirror to practice this part of the technique.

Repeat the washing with the opposite nostril. Always allow the drainage to flow naturally from the nose BEFORE blowing the nose. Blow gently! Always blow gently. If you blow too forcefully, you can experience popping or pain in the ears.

A familiar complaint from first time nose washers is, "It tastes icky!" or "It feels funny when it goes into my throat." But an effective nasal wash technique keeps the solution flowing through the nose, and if this is done correctly none will drip down the throat. It's a learned technique but an easy one to master.

Closing off the throat while you wash is accomplished simply by holding your breath and using the back of your tongue to block the throat. Nose washers have various suggestions to describe their technique: some say make the beginning of the "k" sound without actually saying "k"; this lifts and thickens the tongue in the back. Some say hold your breath, and this works for me, personally. While getting your teeth cleaned, it is a natural reflex to block the back of your throat. It's natural to close the throat in this situation. Others just "do it naturally". Many kids do this without even thinking about it. Over the years, I have found the majority of people understand and find that simply holding your breath while washing works best.

If you do not master this, then you may taste some of the solution in your mouth. This is not harmful, but a bit less effective, and some people find it unpleasant. Just rinse with water and spit. Practice makes perfect.

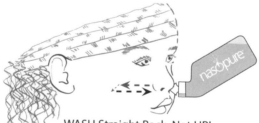

WASH Straight Back, Not UP!

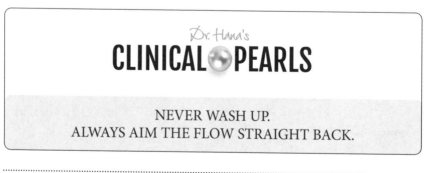

Dr. Hana's
CLINICAL ⬤ PEARLS

NEVER WASH UP.
ALWAYS AIM THE FLOW STRAIGHT BACK.

For Moderate to Severe Congestion

If there is severe congestion on one side, begin by washing, *gently*, the congested side only! As you continue to wash with a hypertonic solution, the swollen membranes will shrink. It may require washing on the congested side several times per day for several days before the nasal passage opens enough to exit the opposite nostril. Once the fluid exits the other side, then it is safe to wash into the unplugged side. Remember, never force it.

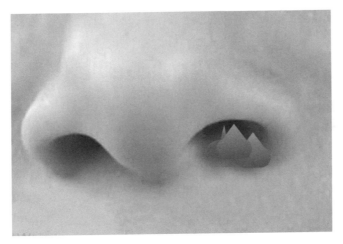

Always wash congested side first and
gently with hypertonic solution

Dr. Hana's
CLINICAL PEARLS

Always wash the congested side **FIRST**.
Always be **GENTLE**.
Always **AVOID** forceful blowing of the nose.

In One Side and Out the Other

··

66 *My mom has been telling everyone she knows about washing her nose. She will ask people, 'Did you know that if you close up your throat and squirt something up one side of your nose it will run out the other side?' Then she proceeds to tell them all about the benefits of nasal washing.* **99**

Sarah R., Miami, Florida

··

A Comfortable Habit

 The salt concentration of the wash solution will vary depending on your comfort level, experience and tolerance. If you experience a burning or stinging sensation, dilute the salt concentration in the solution and then increase the amount of salt as you can tolerate it. Most people increase their tolerance for higher salt concentrations with regular daily nose washing.

A comfortable habit involves a washing system that is easy to perform, feels good, has the right amount of buffered salt, and provides the best results. If you find the right system for you, you are more likely to wash regularly and reap the benefits of this daily practice.

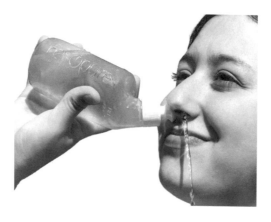

All in One Place: Common Nose Washing Systems

Neti pot:

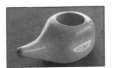

Most modern neti pots are made of clay, opaque plastic or stainless steel. The neti requires bending forward, flexing the neck and rotating the head, so the saline solution can be poured into one nostril. Gravity allows the solution to flow through the nasal passages and out the other nostril. The flow pressure depends on head position in addition to the position and elevation of the neti. The flow also depends upon the amount of obstruction in the nasal tissues, from congestion, a deviated septum or even benign growths on the turbinates *(polyps)*. Neti allows the debris just inside the nose to be introduced into the sinus cavities, with the expectation that it will drain back out again. This position may also allow the solution to enter the ear, causing complaints about water in the ear.

Squeeze bottle:

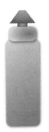

Squeeze bottles are made of plastic with a firm plastic nozzle. Using a squeeze bottle usually requires bending forward and flexing the neck, allowing the solution to be squeezed up into the nostril and sometimes into the sinuses. Flow pressure is determined by how vigorously or gently the bottle is squeezed; the flow from a squeeze bottle must work against gravity. Some squeeze bottles have a straw, some do not. Most encourage a full bottle of solution to be used for each washing. However, these may be awkward to use, placing the bulk of the bottle in your face while you wash.

Nasopure:

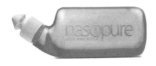

The bottle is made of BPA-free, non-leaching #4 low-density polyethylene plastic with a closeable nozzle. The design of this bottle allows a neutral head position, with no bending forward, flexing of the neck or rotating the head. Nasopure allows solution to be flushed along the nasal floor, the same path that our air follows, then making a U-turn and exiting the opposite nostril. Gravity and the amount of pressure determine the rate of flow. Typically, a full eight ounce bottle of hypertonic solution can last for four to seven days. If several ounces of solution is used, one can actually feel a release, a plunging, so to speak, of the sinus and inner ear cavities without any solution entering the sinus or ear cavity.

Pulsating Mechanical Irrigator:

These electric irrigators require a period of adjustment but once the user is comfortable with this system, it is very effective in cleansing the nasal and sinus tissues. Cost and convenience have been the main hurdles reported to me by my patients. Children and travelers find this system particularly difficult to use.

No More Taco Neck

● ●

66 *The fact that I would be able to flush my nose without contracting 'taco neck', and avoid the chiropractor visit was totally what I needed. I have had rhinoplasty (a nose job) to help control sinusitis and allergies to dust, mold, grass, pollen and most things green and/ or blooming. It was after that surgery that my ENT surgeon instructed me to use saline in order to maintain sinus health now that the cavities had, in essence, been rotor-rootered.*

I have been amazed at the outcome of the saline flushes. I have year-round allergies, which means I spent more time sick than well. Since using the saline solution flushes I have not had any sinusitis for close to ten years. Before the surgery, I had sinusitis continually for five months and no amount of antibiotic could get rid of it. This totally changed my life. 99

Al B, Kansas City, Kansas

● ●

Neti Without Pain in the Neck

66 *I had seen a Neti pot before and thought them to be weird. So I found a nose wash that made sense for me. No turning the head this way and that and whatever else. It just seemed to be an easier way to wash, and easier means I knew my husband would be more apt to use it. We are both at full strength solution and we can both feel a difference. It is taking my husband a little more time, because his head has been clogged for 30 years. He has only taken pills if he got really bad. He has never liked to take pills or vitamins, but he is all about this washing thing; he understands it.* **99**

Janis P., Boston, Massachusetts

All Junk Cleaned Out

66 *I began using a nasal wash last year, it is fantastic! It cleared out major junk! It is so much easier to use than a neti pot!* **99**

Sally K., St. Louis, Missouri

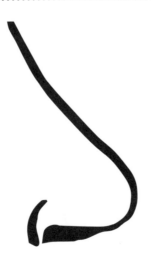

Nasal Irrigation Systems	Neti - Aladdin Style Vessel	Upright Vessel
Neck Position	Bend, Flex and Rotate Neck	Neutral Head and Neck
Pressure Control	Gravity	Gravity and Mild Positive Pressure
Flow Control	Dependent on Angle of Head, Elevation and Position of Vessel, Degree of Nasal Blockage	Limited
Hand Grip	Some lack secure grip	Adequate
Nasal Seal	Variable	Adequate
Tip Design	Some can scratch nasal lining	Adequate
Sinus Suction	None	Partial
Kid Friendly	No	No
Travel Ready	No	No
Solution Level	Difficult to see	Visible
Durability	Clay, Steel or Plastic	Yes
Shower Friendly	Awkward - Potential For Breakage	Variable
Dishwasher Safe	Varies	Yes
Ease of Cleaning	Narrow Tip Difficult To Clean	Yes
Salt Packets	Mix Your Own Solution	10.5 gram weight
Duration Of Salt Supply	Discard Solution After 8 Hours	Manufacturer Recommendations Vary
Salt Composition	Variable, Usually Non-Buffered	Sodium Chloride Sodium Phosphate - Potassium Phosphate
Duration of Mixed Solution	New Mixture For Each Nostril	8 oz Per Washing
Solution Direction	Up Into Sinus Cavity	Straight Back

Squeeze bottle with billow or straw	**Pulsatile Irrigation**	**NASOPURE**
Bend and Flexed Neck	Neutral Head and Neck	Neutral Head and Neck
Positive Pressure, Against Gravity	Mechanical	Gravity and Positive Pressure
Adequate	Mechanical	User Controls Flow, From Small Squirts to Continuous Flushing
Adequate	Easy	Ergonomically Comfortable
Adequate	Adequate	Complete Seal
Good	Good	Safe, Comfortable
None, Floods sinuses	None	Strong Fluid Flush Along Nasal Floor, "Draws" Mucus and Debris Out Of Sinus Cavity, Encourages Natural Drainage
Variable	No	Comfortable and Easy Enough For 2 Years And Older
Variable	No	Portable Tip Snaps Shut to Prevent Leakage
Varies With Different Systems	Visible	Visible
Yes	Unknown	BPA Free, #4 Low-Density Polyethylene, Non-Leaching
Adequate, If Premixed	No	Yes
Yes	No	Yes
Straws Difficult To Clean	N/A	Yes
Variable, Most Less Than 2 gram weight	5 gram weight	3.75 gram weight
Single Packet per 8 oz, Single Use	38 Packets, 1 Month Supply	Discard Hypertonic Solution After 7 Days
Sodium Chloride:Sodium Bicarbonate mix, 2-3% buffered	Sodium Chloride, Sodium Bicarbonate, Xylitol, Potassium Chloride, Calcium Chloride	Sodium Chloride, Sodium Bicarbonate, 33% buffered
8 oz Per Washing	Single Use	Hypertonic Solution Can Last 7 Days
Up Into Sinus Cavity	Up Into Sinus Cavity	Straight Back, Encourages Sinus Drainage

The Dangers of Neti Pot Use—Fact or Fiction?

I have been touting the benefits of nasal cleansing for decades and am a firm believer that washing the personal filter, your nose, makes great sense. The overuse of antibiotics, contributing to increased antibiotic resistant 'superbugs' causes 23,000 deaths in the United States annually. It is vitally important that we carefully limit the use of antibiotics in our daily lives and nasal cleansing is a proven preventative.

Unfortunately, but understandably, these facts are quickly forgotten when faced with the frightening stories of the deaths of two people in 2011, who succumbed to an infection of the brain (primary amoebic meningoencephalitis - PAM) originating from water contaminated by an amoeba used in a neti pot.

Naegleria fowleri is a free-living amoeba that lives and thrives in warm, freshwater ponds, lakes, streams, canals and hot springs. This amoeba primarily affects swimmers who get water up their nose, and mostly in the warm, southern states in the US. In fact, more than half of the infections occurred in just two states. The amoeba travels up the olfactory nerve into the brain causing PAM and is almost always fatal.

Please note that this is a rare occurrence! In the United States from 1962-2012, only 128 cases have been reported to the Centers for Disease Control. In over 50 years only 2 cases were related to a solution made with contaminated water and used in a nasal irrigation device.

These deaths are horrific and regrettable but, by using purified water in a nasal irrigation solution, they are preventable.

I would refer anyone with concerns to the Centers for Disease Control and Prevention website (http://www.cdc.gov/) for complete information on this subject. As a physician and a nasal washer, I recommend always using distilled or purified water to mix a nasal wash solution. This solves the contamination problem easily for those concerned about contracting PAM via a nasal irrigation device.

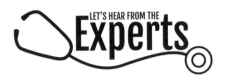

LET'S HEAR FROM THE
Experts

Dr. Kelvin Walls is an ear, nose and throat specialist, a diplomat of the American Board of Otolaryngology. For over two decades he has consulted on both adults and children with nose, sinus and ear woes. His unique approach to treating these problems has encouraged and empowered his patients to actively participate in their medical care. Who better to understand the beneficial effects of nasal washing than an ENT surgeon?

Direct From the Surgeon

I am putting myself out of business because of my recommendations for nasal irrigation. Increased use has mitigated my patients' nasal, ear and throat complaints as much as any new surgical technique or medical therapy. In my opinion, most otolaryngologists are very comfortable prescribing the use of irrigation after surgery. In the past I suggested the use of nasal irrigation for its effectiveness in removing dead tissue, which essentially helps clear a patient's nose after nasal and/or sinus surgery. I have found that the anxiety and stress associated with post-operative recovery can make many patients unreceptive to the trial and benefit of nasal irrigation. Therefore, I now recommend nasal washing before surgery, when they are more open and amenable to understanding and trying a treatment method that is new to them.

Almost immediately after I began suggesting that pre-op patients use nasal irrigation, I noticed that my patients who washed before surgery were dropping off of my surgery schedule. They stated that they were "getting over" their symptoms and their condition had dramatically improved. My first instinct was to attribute this decline in surgery numbers to the patients' reluctance to have surgery. But after a closer look into why these patients improved, I found that nasal cleansing was the key. Patients who washed before (or as it turned out, instead of) surgery were having success treating some of their symptoms for the first time ever. I now teach nasal washing as a frontline therapy for all my patients who have sinus issues.

The Ins and Outs of Nasal Washing

One of the joys of encouraging the use of the irrigation is hearing the testimonies of my patients' success with nasal irrigation. After initially introducing the idea and getting reluctant attitudes about trying it, they often are pleasantly surprised at how well they respond to the treatment. It seems that the more chronic the symptoms the more benefit people get from the irrigation.

Usually, with a sense of disbelief, the patients will say, "This has changed my life. I can't believe that it took me this long to find out about this. This is the first time I have been able to go all winter and haven't got a cold. If I did get a cold, it didn't go into a sinus infection or go into my ears."

Kelvin Walls, MD
Otolaryngologist (ENT; Ears, Nose Throat--Head and Neck Surgeon)
Lees Summit, Missouri

Chapter 6

Dr. Hana's Nasopure

 The magic is in the mix, and the comfort is in the design. Comfort is definitely the key to good results. If you offer someone a wash system that is comfortable, they will actually use it and benefit. That is why I recommend my patented design, Dr. Hana's Nasopure Nasal Wash System. I want to be 100% clear, with full disclosure, that Nasopure is my baby. I *am* biased. But I honestly don't care whether you wash your nose with my product or something else, as long as you *wash your nose every day*!

I have been recommending nasal washing for decades, at first with neti. I started with teaching two-year-olds how to use a neti pot and that was a real adventure! But my patients are the ones who taught me the reasons why they didn't like washing their noses. They told me what was keeping them from washing daily, or at least at the first sign of congestion. I tried many systems, first intuitively knowing, and then personally experiencing the benefits of flushing straight back instead of up. After researching the literature and evaluating the products available around the world it was apparent to me that it was time to develop my own system. A system even my two-year-old patients could use.

I want you to imagine, for a moment, that you have come to my office for medical care. You express concern because you have been prescribed a nasal steroid (by another practitioner) and although it is working, you now have developed nose bleeds. You also share with me your concerns about the long terms effects as well as the cost of the steroid medication.

I review your medical history with you, I conduct a physical exam, and now we are ready to learn from each other. We review your diet, efforts at environmental controls, and daily hygiene habits. We talk about how you can decrease your toxic load by improving your diet, drinking more water, using fewer chemicals on your skin, and controlling for dust mites. These changes, if incorporated into your life, may indeed reduce the need for the steroids. But when I propose that you wash your nose as part of daily hygiene, you reply, "You want me to do *what*, Doctor?!"

Yes, I want you to wash your nose. However, I wouldn't ask you to do something so unfamiliar without providing you with the right tools or the technique to use them.

Most people who wash their nose for the first time assume they must tilt their head up or down or twist it. *No.* With Nasopure, you keep your head straight, keeping your neck in line with the rest of your spine. I have noticed, personally and by listening to my patients, that when washing with an upright head position, people do not experience the uncomfortable sensation of drowning, head filling with water, or any pressure. The goal is to have an enjoyable and satisfying experience, not an uncomfortable one. And nose washing, when done correctly, feels soothing and refreshing, as it should.

If you follow the instructions carefully and apply just a bit of practice, you will soon be enjoying your nose washes like a pro.

The Nasopure Effect

There is a technique to using Dr. Hana's Nasopure bottle, a technique backed up by scientific principles.

Some nasal wash systems claim to wash out your sinuses. But the Nasopure system washes your nose, and in doing so, encourages your sinuses to drain free and naturally. This is called the "Nasopure Effect." Successfully washing the nose, clearing the tiny cilia so they can move effectively again, and using a law of physics called *Bernoulli's Principle* creates the most simple, safe and soothing daily wash possible.

Have you ever noticed how a swiftly moving river draws slower streams into its flow? This is Bernoulli's Principle in action. Bernoulli noticed that as fluid flows more quickly through narrow areas, the pressure within the fluid actually decreases. The faster the flow, the lower the pressure. It is why we see small streams pulled into the swiftly moving flow of large rivers.

Imagine your nose, with Nasopure flowing through, is the river you create each time you wash. Your sinuses are stagnant ponds with small outlets allowing them to drain into the nose. When the saline solution flows past these outlets it creates a low pressure stream that draws out the contents of the sinus cavities just like a swiftly moving river would drain a small pond. And the best part of Nasopure: you control the speed of flow, so you control the pressure differential!

When sinuses and ears are inflamed, you may want to squeeze gently on your Nasopure bottle so you don't irritate tender tissues. Other times, you may want to create a rapidly moving stream of saline that is more aggressive in drawing out the sinuses contents, keeping them open and less likely to become infected. You have control.

But for Bernoulli's Principle to work, you need to direct the flow of solution across the floor of the nasal cavity so it can flow past the sinus openings, creating the pressure differential that drains the sinus contents. If you shoot your solution up instead of back then you may be aiming directly at the openings to the sinuses and the ears. It is as though you are directing the river directly into the pond's outlet - a situation that not only blocks the outward flow, but also can cause transient discomfort as pressure is forced into tiny spaces. And that is exactly why we have designed the Nasopure bottle to encourage flow in the most effective direction.

Not everyone may be familiar with Bernoulli and his principle, but we can all benefit from the science that stands behind the unique design of the Nasopure bottle. Read the instructions, practice your technique, and visualize a swiftly moving river of pure saline flowing past the sinus ponds, drawing out their contents and releasing them as the river flows along the floor of the nose. Finally, take a deep breath, and enjoy the sensation of a clear nose and open sinuses. So good!

Thank you Mr. Bernoulli.

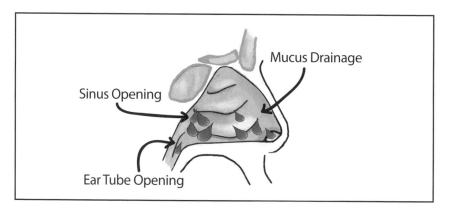

#1 Nasal Passages Filled with Mucus

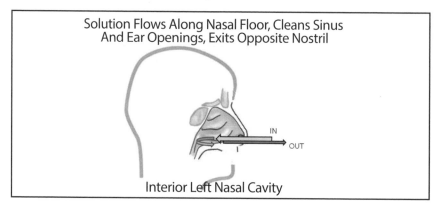

#2 Solution Flushes Along Nasal Floor

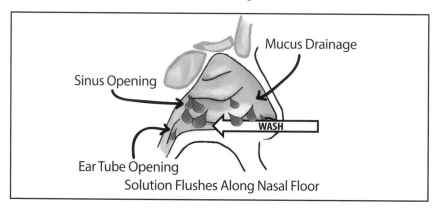

#3 Nasopure Wash

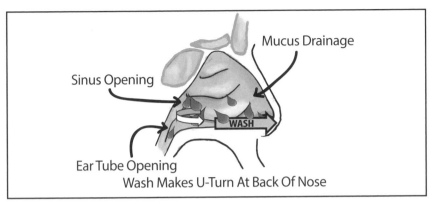

#4 Nasopure Wash, Makes U-Turn

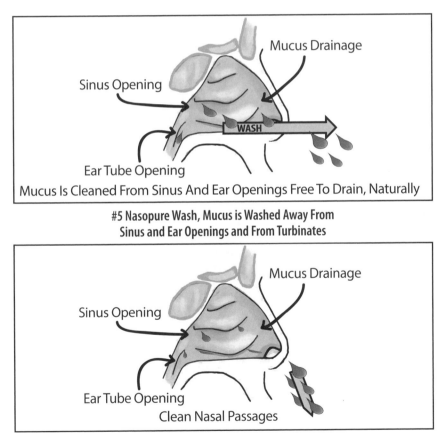

#5 Nasopure Wash, Mucus is Washed Away From Sinus and Ear Openings and From Turbinates

#6 Nasopure Wash, Nasal Passages Are Cleaned

Salt. Is it Kosher? Does it matter?

The salt components in Nasopure are not common table salt. These are pharmaceutical grade, fine granules of sodium chloride and sodium bicarbonate combined in a ratio which is scientifically supported to be the most effective and comfortable. The buffering added by the inclusion of the sodium bicarbonate can augment healing of tissues. This mixture is free of trace minerals and due to the tiny granule size, it dissolves instantly and is soothing to the membranes.

Nasopure Studied for Effectiveness

After many of my patients were using the Nasopure system, I decided to document their objective responses to using this device so I designed a formal study. This study was approved by the University Of Missouri Investigational Review Board in 2004. This board's function is to ensure that all approved medical studies are both safe and scientific. Regular Nasopure users responded to questions retrospectively (after they washed regularly for a minimum of one month). The results confirmed what other studies also found. Overall, patients reported that their symptoms were improved or eliminated and that their medication use was reduced. Overall satisfaction was clearly demonstrated.

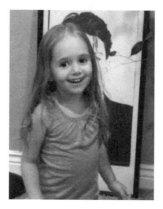

CLINICAL PEARLS

Dr. Hana's

> If everyone is offered a quick fix, everyone may try it, but few will continue to use it unless it is comfortable and convenient.

Detailed Instructions on Using the Nasopure System

Washing your nose with any nasal irrigation system is most effective when done correctly. Read the detailed, step-by-step instructions that come with the system you choose to use. I suggest following my instructions and allowing three days to perfect the technique, although many people feel the results immediately. It may take practice.

Adults may need to get over fearful past experiences. Some adults remember being pushed into a swimming pool and thinking they might drown. Often adults will assume that the water will go upward and cause an uncomfortable experience, but this is not true. Some may have tried another wash system and fear the same uncomfortable results. It is interesting to note that most children can learn this technique almost immediately because they do not have the fear that comes from negative past experiences.

Note: Specific instructions for teaching children how to wash their nose can be found in Chapter 7.

The best time to incorporate washing into your daily routine is in the shower or after brushing your teeth while leaning over the sink. The key is to integrate the habit with an already established routine.

CARING FOR YOUR SYSTEM

Wash your Nasopure bottle and tip using mild dish soap and warm water. Rinse well. Your bottle may be disinfected periodically with one to two drops of bleach in a soapy solution. Wash, rinse and dry thoroughly. Bottles are dishwasher safe on the top rack.

MIXING YOUR NASOPURE SOLUTION

✓ Add Nasopure buffered salt packet to bottle (see Solution Guide) and fill bottle with purified, distilled or previously boiled water.

✓ Twist cap onto bottle; close by pushing down on tip. Mix.

✓ Rinse cap after each use.

✓ Discard remaining hypertonic solution after one week. Isotonic solution should be discarded daily.

✓ Wash bottle and tip. Dry thoroughly before mixing new solution.

✓ Always store your solution at room temperature.

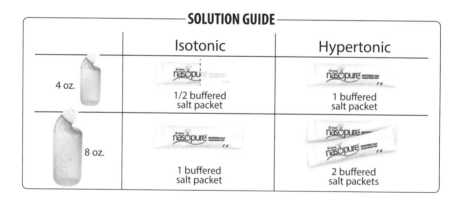

SOLUTION GUIDE	Isotonic	Hypertonic
4 oz.	1/2 buffered salt packet	1 buffered salt packet
8 oz.	1 buffered salt packet	2 buffered salt packets

HOW OFTEN SHOULD YOU WASH?

✓ For prevention - Use once per day or after exposure to irritants.

✓ For mild to moderate congestion or discharge - Use twice daily.

✓ For moderate to severe congestion, discharge or infection - Use three or four times daily.

USING NASOPURE

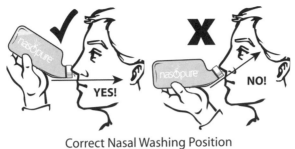

Correct Nasal Washing Position

✓ Most people prefer washing while in the shower or standing over a sink.

✓ Keep your head straight and look forward. There is no need to bend your neck.

✓ Place bottle tip into one nostril and point the tip toward the back of your throat, not pointing to the eyes. DO NOT POINT TIP UPWARD. Do not confuse the position of the bottle with the tip - if the bottle is aimed at the throat, the tip will then be incorrectly aimed upward.

✓ Seal nostril with bottle tip.

✓ Block the back of the throat by holding your breath while gently squeezing the bottle. Learning how to block your throat may take practice and will prevent the solution from reaching the mouth, resulting in a salty taste. If this occurs, it is not harmful.

✓ SQUEEZE BOTTLE GENTLY, flushing solution along the nasal floor, allowing it to make a U-turn at the back of your throat and exiting the opposite nostril. You may experience a mild burning sensation with the first use. This is normal, not harmful and will disappear with repeated use.

✓ Switch to other nostril and repeat.

✓ Allow your nose to drain naturally. Exhale through nose with mouth closed.

✓ BLOW NOSE GENTLY.

✓ DO NOT BLOCK OR PINCH OPPOSITE NOSTRIL WHEN WASHING OR BLOWING.

✓ To allow any trapped solution to drain, bend forward from the waist and gently rotate your head from side to side.

MODERATE TO SEVERE CONGESTION

- ✓ If there is congestion on one side, gently wash on the congested side only! As you continue to wash with a hypertonic solution the swollen membranes will shrink. For example, if the left side is blocked, wash gently on the left side only, not expecting the flush to exit the opposite nostril. Repeat two to four times per day. If the blockage begins to open and the solution exits the right side, then it is safe to begin flushing both nostrils.

- ✓ Washing only on the congested side may be required for several days before swollen passages shrink, allowing solution to exit the opposite nostril. Never force it!

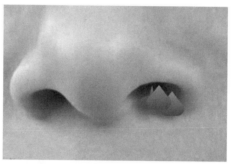

Always wash congested side first and gently with hypertonic solution

CHILDREN

Never wash for a child! Never force a child to wash! Make it fun!

See Chapter 7 for specific, age-appropriate instructions, how to teach your child to nose-blow, and what to do if your child is afraid of water.

If your child has recurrent ear or sinus problems, is disabled, or has difficulty tolerating the wash, consult your doctor.

- ✓ Always begin with isotonic solution and advance as your child tolerates.

- ✓ Use 1/2 packet of Nasopure buffered salt in the Little Squirt *to go*® bottle and purified, distilled, or previously boiled water.

- ✓ Help make sure your child is holding the bottle correctly and encourage them to squeeze gently, give them the control and power. Give them kudos for *any* attempt!
- ✓ Encourage your child to gently squeeze a small amount of solution (approximately one teaspoon) into each nostril. Young children will automatically block the back of their throat.
- ✓ Encourage the child to blow their nose gently.
- ✓ NOTE: Allow your child to watch videos of other kids washing, then allow them to watch you wash first, while they play with the bottle, getting accustomed to the feel of the spray. You can find some good videos to share at www.nasopure.com. Make it fun!

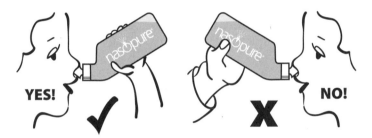

How Often Should Your Child Wash?

- ✓ Once per day at a minimum for prevention.
- ✓ Twice per day if any symptoms are present or after exposure to any irritants.
- ✓ Three to four times per day if infection is present.
- ✓ Wash immediately after potential exposure to airborne illness or any irritants.

Anyone can learn how to wash his or her nose. Of course, there are challenges. You have to incorporate the process into your daily hygiene routine, much like brushing your teeth. Another downside is that the process is not attractive or sexy, but then neither is brushing your teeth! The process is so simple and the cost so affordable, some people assume washing can't be as effective as a pill.

Avoiding the Pain

66 *I saw an ear, nose, and throat specialist to understand why my head was always congested, in spite of taking decongestants and steroid nasal and asthma medications. An MRI showed my sinuses to be completely clogged, so he wanted to wash them out by sticking a syringe through the bony tissue in my nose. In the meantime, I began nasal rinsing. When the doctor washed out my left sinus, nothing came out. It had already been cleared by using Nasopure, so he didn't have to do the right one.* **99**

Fred M, San Carlos, California

Clean Nose Kid

66 *I read about Nasopure in Parents Magazine. It sounded like the perfect thing for my five-year-old son who has been having a really rough time with his runny nose due to allergies. After about four to five days I noticed that his nose was much more clear! I would and will definitely recommend this! Thank you guys very much!* **99**

Jessica C, Napoleon, Ohio

Possible Side Effects of Nasal Washing

1. Burning sensation
   - ✓ Often related to mucosal inflammation.
   - ✓ Will subside with continued washing.
   - ✓ Will be less likely to occur if the salinity is either too much or too little, or not buffered appropriately.

2. Ear popping

   ✓ Technique: be sure to point the solution towards the back of the throat. If congested, the shrinking of the swollen ear opening allows air to percolate upward, hence "ear popping." This is a good sign because it means the Eustachian tube is opening up. The ear popping will subside with subsequent washings.

   ✓ Following washing: do not blow vigorously. This can cause air to be forced backwards into the ear tube.

   ✓ Eustachian tube dysfunction already exists: if the ear already contains fluid, ear popping will occur. Just keep washing gently, blow gently, and this will resolve as the Eustachian tube becomes clear. Hypertonic solution works best for this particular situation.

   ✓ Forceful washing can cause a transient popping of the ears. DO NOT FORCE!

3. Water drips unexpectedly from the nose after washing

   ✓ Technique: the solution is directed upward into the sinuses where it can become trapped, unexpectedly causing solution to flow out later when the sinus ostia decongest and open. Hold the bottle as directed, with the bottom of the bottle almost pointing toward the ceiling, tip pointed straight back, at the level of the neck, ensuring the flush goes along the nasal floor.

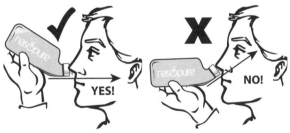

Correct Nasal Washing Position

   ✓ Swollen mucous membranes: The solution finds a hidden pocket in the swollen membrane and gets trapped. The saline decongests the nose, shrinking the swollen membranes and the leftover solution drains out. This will resolve once the tissues heal.

✓ Advice: if this is a problem for you, try this technique: after washing, and after allowing the natural drainage to exit from your nostrils, blow very gently without blocking one nostril closed. Then, slowly, bend from your waist, and allow your arms to dangle freely, relaxing there for a moment. Then, very slowly and gently turn your head so that your chin approaches or touches your shoulder. Repeat for other side. This will allow any trapped solution to drain naturally.

Important Considerations

✓ *Never block the opposite nostril to prevent solution from draining freely.*

✓ Do not use immediately before bed, as water may drip from your nose for several minutes after washing.

✓ If you experience burning or stinging, change the strength of the saline solution. You could be using too little salt, too much salt or not enough buffering.

✓ Never force anyone else to wash.

✓ Do not lie down while using any nasal irrigation system.

✓ Do not microwave plastic bottles, ever.

✓ Wash the nose prior to using prescribed nasal sprays.

✓ Be gentle. Never force!

✓ Blow very gently after allowing the solution to drain naturally.

✓ Each bottle is intended for a single user, like a toothbrush.

✓ Discard solution after one week if using hypertonic solution, and remix a fresh batch after washing the bottle and cap. If using isotonic solution, mix a fresh batch daily. Rinse the cap after each use.

✓ Use warm solution to wash with. Cold solution can be uncomfortable. Never use hot water. Some people enjoy room temperature water and find it refreshing.

✓ Store solution at room temperature.

✓ Check out www.nasopure.com for more information or contact me for questions regarding your nasal washing experience.

✓ Consult your doctor if symptoms worsen or if you have a significant medical condition.

Dr. Hana's
CLINICAL⬤PEARLS

- Any washing is better than no washing.
- Learning curves vary, so be patient.
- Kids learn easier if at least one parent demonstrates or if they are allowed to watch a video of other kids.
- Washing should always precede any prescription nasal medication.
- It usually takes one to three days to master the art of nasal washing.
- Always begin with isotonic and increase the salinity as tolerated.
- Hypertonic works best.
- Everyone can learn to close their throat while washing; holding your breath seems to work best for most people.
- Senior citizens appreciate the benefits of nose washing.
- Never force anyone to wash.
- If you can stand and brush your own teeth, you can learn how to wash.
- Nose washing is not sexy: neither is a snotty nose.
- Your nose feels refreshed and soothed after washing.
- Washing your nose represents a long-term hygiene strategy aimed at prevention.
- Do Not Blow Vigorously. Never. Ever.

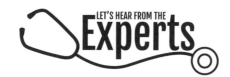

Special Section: Let's Hear From The Experts, In This Case: Parents!

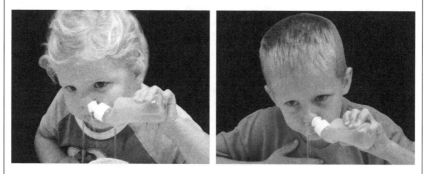

My Nasopure story began several years ago. I had heard of nasal irrigation from a couple of sources but did not know of any easy way to accomplish rinsing your nose with a "salty" solution. My introduction to nose washing was very informal, probably during a visit to our family physician during the cold and flu season. At that time I was a little apprehensive about how to correctly irrigate my nasal passages. However, I mixed up the solution as the doctors had instructed and took a stab, or rather a squirt, at "hosing my nose". To my amazement, I got it right on my first try. Didn't cough, didn't drown and I was overwhelmed with a sense of cleansing in my nasal passages. From that point forward, I was sold.

Since that time, I have had a few colds, sinus infections and such, but washing my nose has lessened or eliminated symptoms, and in general, has helped reduce the duration of my nasal related issues. As my wife and I have discovered, one of the best ways to learn and perfect the technique is to use a mirror when doing it. The visual feedback you get from the mirror will guide you on how much pressure to exert on squeezing the bottle when irrigating your nose. Another thing that we've also discovered is that doing it in the shower helps too.

Our first-born child Matthew has experienced allergic-type symptoms to common indoor and outdoor allergens (i.e. dust, pollen, grasses). Fairly early in his life, around two years old, Matthew became a somewhat frequent user of an oral antihistamine. This medication, though improving Matthew's quality of breathing, was not what we wanted for Matthew long term. When Matthew was about three and a half years old, we began introducing him slowly to washing his nose. My wife and I would demonstrate how and explain why it would clean out our noses and help us breathe better too. For Matthew, the best place for learning was in the shower. We would make a game of it see who could rinse out the best boogers first. Matthew continued to use Zyrtec on occasion as washing on a regular basis did not happen right away. But with careful persistence, Matthew became a regular washer, just like brushing his teeth daily. Now at five and a half years of age, he takes no medications for allergy related symptoms. Matthew's younger sister Rachel, wanting to be just like big brother, took her first shot at nose washing before she was three years old. She saw Matthew at the sink one day with the bottle and decided she had to try it. Rachel does not suffer from allergic symptoms as severe as Matthew's but she still wanted to be like big brother. And like big brother she was. In fact she is a natural. She picked it up easier than Matthew and they both are true nose washers. I don't know if this is a coincidence, but Rachel took her first swimming lessons after learning to flush water into her nose when she was three and very quickly became at ease while going under water. It is my belief that learning to do hold your breath and closing off your throat has helped her advance in swimming class at a much faster pace.

One final note: Our family began using isotonic buffered salt when we started our journey. And I would certainly encourage isotonic mixture in the beginning. As we became more comfortable, we have made it all the way up to hypertonic solution. It is a little more intense, but boy does it do a thorough cleaning of your nasal passages! I am so thankful that I have become acquainted with nasal washing. My nose and my family's noses certainly appreciate it.

Sincerely, Michael Griffith and family, Missouri

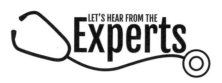

The Right Cure for Many Ills

As a rural GP and Emergency Medicine Attending Physician, I've seen the gamut of medical conditions over the past fifteen years, and have explored a myriad of options for most of them. Since fortuitously stumbling upon Dr. Hana's Nasopure I've recommended it for no small variety of conditions, and have found it particularly successful in treating nasal and sinus congestion in all of its varied forms - viral coryza (head colds), allergic and irritant congestion, and both viral and bacterial sinusitis. I've certainly recommended neti pots and salt water inhalations in the past, but had found both patient acceptance and efficacy sadly problematic. The idea of pouring the contents of a tiny teapot into one's nose was a difficult sell to the non-Indian patient, and even to those who'd grown up culturally accepting such a measure! The plastic Nasopure bottle however was an object that looks more-or-less familiar to the majority of my patients, and was (rather surprisingly to me) quite readily accepted - even by young children and teenagers!

Clinically, the results have been most gratifying - with the result that something I'd initially had to "sell" somewhat to the patients has now become familiar and accepted through word-of-mouth alone in our small town! As respiratory illnesses often begin in the nose and upper airways, it's seemed to me as if early treatment with nose washing may actually have aborted the progression of colds in some of my patients, along with alleviating the severity of their earliest symptoms. Whether patients are suffering allergic asthma (that triggered by mold, pollens, grasses, dust mites, etc.) or irritant asthma (due to pollution, smog, chemical fumes, etc.), treatment with nasal rinsing has often provided amazing relief of both the upper airway symptoms and the secondarily-triggered asthmatic symptoms of wheeze and chest congestion. It's certainly been a life-saver for a majority of these patients, and has in many cases dramatically reduced their use of not only inhaled steroids but both short and long-acting beta agonists (i.e., salbutamol).

Not surprisingly, I've also had successes with nasal washing in treating chronic post-nasal drip, and occasionally patients have even reported a reduction in snoring as described by their sleep partners. As a practicing physician exposed on a daily basis to all manner of respiratory pathogens, I tend to practice this regimen myself near-religiously at the end of the work day to purge my nostrils of any viruses or bacteria which might be attempting to infect me. Although I've not truly documented my experience, I do feel that this intervention has served me well in helping me to avoid occupational illness despite my high-risk profession.

I would highly recommend both the daily practice of nose washing and Dr. Hana's well-designed little device to anyone with the above-mentioned conditions, or anyone with an interest in nasal health. I strongly feel that it should be a mainstay in the therapeutic repertoire of any ENT physician, pediatrician or general practitioner.

Lawrence W. Klein, MD
Family Practice, Emergency, Integrative and Nutritional Medicine
Squamish, British Columbia, Canada

Easier Than Neti

" *I really like my Nasopure bottle and use it routinely - especially now, in allergy and cold season. It is so much easier to use than a neti pot. I use mine in the shower, so much quicker and no mess! I am purchasing Nasopure kits for Christmas gifts. My hat goes off to Dr. Hana for a great alternative to medicine. The salt packets are so convenient and not as harsh as sea salt. I recommend this system to people of all ages.* **"**

Lindy M, Enfield, Illinois

Ceramic Neti Breaks

" *My granddaughter has lupus, a small brain aneurysm, high blood pressure and sinus problems, so we need Nasopure to help. We recently moved and the sudden change of climate from San Francisco to Arizona's dry climate has set off her sinus problems. Then this morning she was working with her ceramic neti pot, but it broke. She called me to find out how she could get one of yours. So I looked on the bottom of my box and, God bless, your number was there. Thank you for returning my call on a Sunday and getting a Nasopure system sent so quickly.* **"**

Jacqueline O, Prescott, Arizona

Part III

Everybody Has a Nose

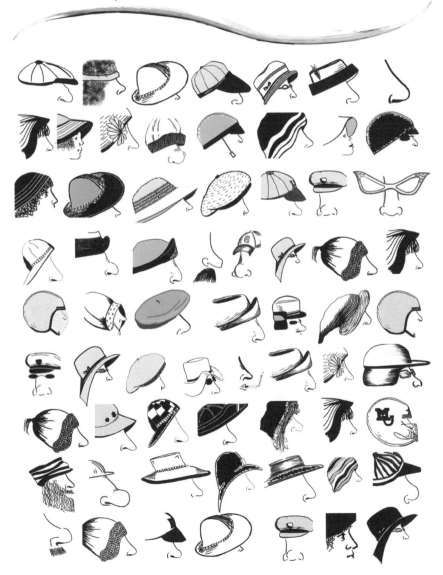

Chapter 7

Infants and Babies
Need Clean Noses

 I have cared for many infants and I know that every healthy infant has simple needs. A baby needs to be well fed, well rested, dressed appropriately, but most important, the baby needs to breathe! Breathing through the nose is a must for any infant to thrive.

A congested nose that needs cleaning is a common problem in babies, but what new parent doesn't have a love/hate relationship with the Big Blue Bulb? It is part of the kit you are given when you come home from the hospital or birth center - along with your new baby, flowers, plants, diapers and a pile of paperwork. And love it or hate it, you've been told that the suction bulb could be important if your baby has a stuffy nose.

I refer to the "blue-bulb-torture" and universally, parents smile and agree it brings up images of a screaming baby and frustrated parents. Why is this so? It is hard (if not impossible) to clean, it doesn't work all that well, and it is just plain uncomfortable for everyone involved.

For the most part, newborns are obligate nose breathers. That means they must breathe through their nose and are only going to switch to mouth breathing when significantly depleted of oxygen. So it is important to keep a newborn's nose clear.

In 2012 the International Journal of Pediatrics published a study with the long title: "It Takes a Mouth to Eat and a Nose to Breathe: Abnormal Oral Respiration Affects Neonates' Oral Competence and Systemic Adaptation." This study explained in their conclusion, "... the nose is more than a simple duct directing air to the lungs. From the very first breath it also services sensory processes that are involved in the regulation of respiration and of general behavior mediated by the mouth (feeding motivation, orientation, and learning based on olfaction). At least in newborn and young mammals, the mouth has been emancipated from any involvement in respiration, leaving it reserved for ingestion, exploration and communication. When incidental nasal obstruction occurs, all these functions are deferred in favor of maintaining air supply to the lungs. This change is far from benign…A first major effect of this competition between respiration and ingestion at the mouth level is a reduced and disorganized sucking performance and a deprivation of sensory inputs to the developing olfactory tracts. It cannot be excluded that the dehydration incurred to oral and lingual mucosae by oral respiration may also affect gustatory abilities."

 Every parent wants their child to be able to eat well, to develop their senses fully, and to breathe easily. Toward this basic nurturing goal, parents may need to clear a tiny nose. But babies' noses are so small, and the tip of the bulb doesn't fit easily into a newborn's, or even an older infant's nostril. Who wants to fight a screaming infant just to get a single drop of mucus out of that teeny tiny tender space?

Mucus, although the most common cause of obstruction, is not the only possible problem encountered by newborn noses. If nasal obstruction is persistent or severe, a visit to the doctor may be wise to rule out something more serious than nasal irritation or a self-limiting virus. But before going to the doctor, parents should clean their baby's congested nose three to four times a day because the problem may be simple mucus or swollen membranes. For the occasional stuffy nose that gets in the way of easy breathing, sleeping, and nursing, parents can learn to clear even a newborn's nose without causing a scene or even making their infant cry. It's all in the technique.

Causes of Infant Congestion

Viral infection - According to the Mayo Clinic, infants may catch six to ten colds each year.

- Allergies (after the first nine to twelve months of age).
- Irritants in the environment.
- Gastroesophageal reflux.
- Enlarged adenoids.
- Normal mucus accumulation.
- Cystic fibrosis or other congenital abnormalities.
- Congenital polyps

First, throw that blue bulb syringe away. After all, it probably has mold growing inside and shouldn't be anywhere near a baby's nose. Avoid using medication to clear an infant's nose - the side effects (hyperactivity or sedation, appetite changes, behavioral changes, thickened secretions) are not worth the questionable benefits. This is especially true for babies younger than three months old. And besides, we know that medicine only treats symptoms, not the cause. Clean the nose first. You and your baby will get better results with a little saline nasal irrigation and gentle aspiration, using a system designed for just this purpose.

There are various baby aspirator designs, some using hand suction, some mouth suction and some are even motorized. Make yourself familiar with the design you choose so you are comfortable enough to keep your baby calm while using it. It should have a soft silicone-like tip that is easy to fit into your baby's nostril. A chamber that traps mucus can isolate the mucus safely. With these features, you can maintain complete control of both placement of the tip and the suction. The pull force can be tested by placing the silicone tip onto the fat pad of your own finger when creating suction. You'll feel a gentle tug. Nothing to be afraid of!

If your baby's mucus is dry or sticky, it is good to thin that mucus before trying to remove it. Put one or two drops of isotonic saline solution in her nose while she is sitting upright with her head higher than her body.

She won't feel so vulnerable in this position. She may not like the taste of that salt water, but it is safe if it does drain into her throat - as long as the drops of saline are given while the baby's head is higher than her chest. After a few minutes, the mucus will be thin enough to suction.

Cradle your baby in your arms, or hold her on your lap facing you. Put the soft nozzle inside her nostril, making a complete seal. Be sure to direct the tip towards her neck, not towards her eyes. Correct placement and direction of the tip will ensure comfort and the most effective results. Now create the suction, and watch the mucus collect. Then repeat the same process in the other nostril. Her nose should now be clear enough to breathe and suck without difficulty. You can repeat this as often as needed while your baby is congested.

This whole process should be gentle and when done correctly, actually feels good to your baby. Don't fight it. If your baby resists vigorously, back off and try again later when you and she are both calm.

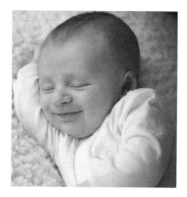

BENEFITS OF INFANT NASAL CLEANSING

✓ Deeper and better sleep.
✓ Normal appetite.
✓ Reduced number of illnesses (ear, asthma, sinus, cough, sore throat).
✓ Hearing not impaired and improved language development.

After a few months, your newborn is no longer tiny and you are not as fearful about doing things "wrong." Your baby is more active, able to move around and squirm with strength, even moving on to crawling and toddling all over the place. But the runny noses don't go away; as a matter of fact, they may increase as you interact with other families and your child's immune system begins to build defenses against common viruses and other irritants. At some point your baby will learn how to blow his nose into a tissue (see page 140 on teaching your child to blow her nose), and by the age of two he may be able to self-use a nose washing system just right for his size. In the meantime, you still must provide help with congested noses - more help than a quick swipe of a tissue as they toddle by on their way to the next adventure!

It is more important than ever to continue washing your child's nose as he toddles through the first two years. Children whose parents include nose washing as a regular part of good hygiene have reduced risk of ear infections, night coughs, and asthma. These children have improved language and listening skills, they sleep better and breathe better. They spread fewer germs picked up in daycare and react less to allergens. More importantly, they need antibiotics less than children who don't wash their nose regularly.

The toddler years are the perfect time to teach skills that can last a lifetime. Make the nose wash a part of bath-time. Let him play with it along with his other bath toys and then do a quick rinse of his nose with clean saline before getting out of the tub. A child that has had his nose washed since he was an infant will not balk at learning to wash it himself as soon as he is able. It's as easy as learning to brush his teeth! Maybe even easier.

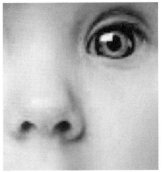

Chapter 8

Children

Kids and Colds - The Seemingly Endless Connection

 Kids get colds. On average, kids get anywhere from three to nine colds each year, depending on their age, number of siblings in the home, and their social interactions. While these viral infections are helpful because they build immunities, in children younger than preschool-age colds can lead to complications such as ear, chest and sinus infections. There are ways to minimize the number of sick days and the miseries of the cold and flu season.

The U.S. Food and Drug Administration frequently updates their advisory stating that over-the-counter (OTC) cough and cold medicines should not be given to infants and children. The cut-off age for safe use of OTC medications has been revised more than once, so prudent caution is wise. Side effects of these products and the risk of overdoses are serious concerns. Washing the nose, a more holistic alternative, has few minor side effects *and* does not contribute to the growing problem of antibiotic resistance.

Several recent studies involving children support both my clinical experience and what many other doctors already know. Nasal washing in children reduces the number of colds and other respiratory infections. Those who irrigate with saline use fewer medications, including fever reducers, decongestants and antibiotics. The nasal wash groups also face shorter illnesses and fewer missed school days. This news finally supports a common-sense approach I have valued since the early days of my medical practice: "If it's dirty, wash it!"

Children and Ears

 Americans spend billions of dollars each year treating ear problems in children; much of it on doctor visits, drugs and surgery. Ear infections are the number one reason children visit a doctor's office, and the number of children coming in with ear infections has risen over the past decade. There are several reasons for this, including bottle-feeding, increased allergies, greater pollution, more children in daycare, and exposure to cigarette smoke. Interestingly, boys develop infections in the ears more often than girls do, and it is not clear why.

Children in general seem to experience far more ear infections then adults, and this is because their Eustachian tubes are immature (see figure on page 31). Infants and children have a more horizontal Eustachian tube without gravity to assist in drainage. It is also much shorter and collapses more easily compared to an adult tube; the opening in the throat is more rounded, making it easier for secretions to find their way up into the middle ear. Additionally, babies tend not to swallow when they are asleep (they drool), and less swallowing means less ventilation of the middle ear. All of these differences result in a buildup of negative pressure, which causes pain and leads to restless nights.

Anyone who has had difficulty clearing their ears after flying in an airplane, or anyone who has had the congestion of a cold that "clogged" their ears knows how Eustachian tube dysfunction feels. Children with chronic nasal congestion can feel this way all the time. These children think the world always sounds muffled and it is no surprise that they cannot speak clearly. The most common causes of Eustachian tube dysfunction are allergies and respiratory infections. Traditionally doctors have given antihistamines to dry up secretions and decongestants to clear the passages. However, the side effects of these two medications can be problematic, especially in children.

Molly was brought into my clinic by her mother. Both Molly's mom and kindergarten teacher were concerned that she was not paying attention in class. A quick screen in the office indicated a "conductive hearing loss." Mom wanted to avoid medications if possible, so she agreed to try nasal rinsing. Soon Molly was washing like a pro, and two weeks later the repeat hearing test was normal. A simple and safe approach resolved her problem.

Hearing is one of the most important windows to a child's world. Through good hearing, a child learns language skills and an appreciation for the world around him or her. If you are concerned about your child's ability to hear well, speak to your physician. If the problem is chronic congestion or infections, ask about nasal washing.

Adenoids and tonsils are lymph tissues that normally enlarge as a child ages, peaking in size during elementary school years and beginning to shrink just before puberty. The adenoids are situated in the upper throat, in the back part of the nose, right next to the Eustachian tube opening. The tonsils are lower in the throat. These tissues will remain enlarged if constantly irritated, aggravated and stimulated by recurrent infections or allergies. Chronically enlarged tissues prevent the Eustachian tube's normal drainage, which can contribute to recurrent ear infections.

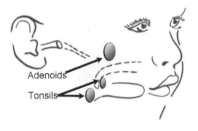

For years, doctors would automatically prescribe antibiotics when any fluid was found in the middle ear, especially in children. If the fluid persisted, they would recommend surgical placement of drainage ports, *PE tubes*, in the eardrum - a man-made exit for the fluid. These tubes do not correct the original problem, but they do allow the fluid to drain out the ear canal if the Eustachian tube is blocked. More recently, the Academy of Pediatrics acknowledged that routine antibiotics and PE tubes may not be the best approach and has now released new recommendations. A watch and wait approach to most ear infections is the newest guideline, but as in the past, it is up to each physician to decide on the necessity of using antibiotics and/or surgery.

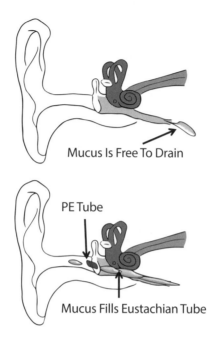

Mucus Is Free To Drain

PE Tube

Mucus Fills Eustachian Tube

These recommendations will hopefully contribute to a decrease in the overuse of antibiotics and a reduction in bacterial resistance. Using fewer medications will reduce the development of adverse drug reactions as well. Sometimes these medications are warranted, but I recommend a first line treatment that is much safer and often more effective in addressing the core issue as compared to medication: nasal washing with hypertonic buffered salt water.

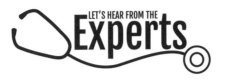

Antibiotic overuse is a particular concern. Many children with nasal disease seem to become "antibiotic-dependent," that is, their symptoms seem to be relieved while taking antibiotics, but then relapse shortly after the treatment course ends. A new antibiotic is then started, and the cycle then repeats itself over and over, sometimes for many months.

Michael Cooperstock, MD, MPH
Pediatric Infectious Disease
University of Missouri, Columbia, Medical Center

Tips to reduce ear infections

- Breastfeed instead of bottle-feed.
- Avoid exposing your child to cigarette smoke.
- Adjust living environment for fewer allergens.
- Provide healthy unprocessed foods for fewer allergies.
- Avoid daycare if your child is younger than two years old.
- Keep the nose clean.
- Avoid medications that dry and thicken the mucus, such as antihistamines.
- Maintain hydration, avoid sugary juices (teach your children to drink water).
- Treat GERD (Gastroesophageal Reflux) if it is present.
- Apply warmed moist compresses to the outer ear for 20 minutes every few hours.
- Work with your child's medical provider so that your collaborative efforts will bring about the most effective and least invasive solutions.
- If your child is getting worse, see your medical provider!

School Days

 When school starts at the end of each summer parents may be relieved to have their kids back in the classroom, but they are also aware that this is when everyone starts getting sick again. Schools are wonderful breeding grounds for viruses and some of this illness is inevitable, even desirable. After all, fighting viruses is how we build immunities, so some illness is actually good for our health. But try to tell that to a sick kid, or the mother of a sick kid! Taking measures to prevent sickness is always a good idea, and there is much you can do to keep your kids healthy through the fall and winter months. Wholesome nutritious foods and adequate restorative sleep are common sense measures that go a long way towards fighting infections.

Teaching children to wash their hands is probably the most popular health measure. Reinforce this healthy habit by asking your kids to clean their hands regularly when you are with them. Make sure they wash before eating any food, even snacks. While you are teaching your children to wash their hands, it's a good idea to teach them to wash their nose also. Our grandmothers knew the health values of salt water and we have grown to appreciate their wisdom. Learning to wash can be fun for kids, especially when they are healthy.

When a child develops cold symptoms, I encourage parents to manage that cold with twice-a-day nasal washing; it is a natural decongestant and soothes inflamed mucous membranes. There are no side effects to the simple combination of rest, fluids, washing the virus particles out of the nose and patiently allowing the body to heal itself.

Dr. Hana's
CLINICAL PEARLS

The secret to teaching children how to wash their nose
is a slow introduction, giving the child all of the control,
praising them frequently for little steps, and asking
them to demonstrate their technique for others.

Before we get into the nuts and bolts of keeping your kids' noses clean and clear, here are some very important things to keep in mind:

✓ Many children can prevent or reduce chronic nasal/sinus problems by regular nasal washing.

✓ It can be challenging to get a child to practice healthful habits.

✓ Do not expect daily use.

✓ The goal is for children to become skillful and comfortable in washing.

✓ Use as needed to avoid illness after exposure to those who may be ill or as daily prevention for chronic symptoms.

✓ Children are more likely to use a formula that is free of additives because it does not burn.

✓ Use a child-sized bottle.

✓ Use a solution, either isotonic or hypertonic, that does not burn.

✓ Offer the child complete control. Empower your child.

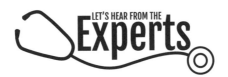
LET'S HEAR FROM THE
Experts

I have confidence when I recommend nasal wash for my patients. With all the ear, nose, and throat issues that children experience, I am certain that simply washing the nasal lining has great benefits without risk. My patients quickly learn the simple technique and I find that they use fewer medications and experience both fewer symptoms and fewer infections. Nasal washing has proven to be tolerable, safe, convenient and effective for my pediatric patients. Maintenance of nasal and sinus health with the modernized version of an ancient technique of nasal irrigation just makes sense.

Marcella R. Bothwell, MD
Otolaryngology, Pediatric Otolaryngology, San Diego, California

No More Sinus Surgeries

66 *Our daughter Madelyn has been using the Nasopure system for almost a year. At the age of three she was facing her second sinus surgery. We have had much success and she has only had one round of antibiotics this year! I hope you know how much we appreciate you and Nasopure. We attribute Nasopure to saving Madelyn's life. She had such severe infections that she began to lose her hair, drastically lost weight, and had multiple admissions for failure to thrive. One night in the hospital I was reading blogs on the Internet and came upon one about Nasopure. By the time that we found your product, Mady had been admitted to the hospital with a potassium level of 2.5. Needless to say, two years later, she is a happy and healthy four-year-old. I feel like we need the Nasopure to keep her healthy. Thank you for saving our sweet girl!* **99**

Sara W, Chicago, Illinois

Dr. Hana's
CLINICAL PEARLS

Be a good example; washing can be a family affair.

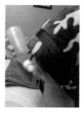

Teaching Your Child to Wash

 Four-year-old Brianna had ongoing ear and sinus problems, requiring multiple medications to control her allergy symptoms. I introduced Brianna to washing her nose by encouraging her to fill the bottle with warm water and just play with it during her daily bath. This helped her get the feel of the pressure needed to spray water out the tip. Next, we suggested to her that if she tried to squirt just a bit of water in her nose, it would help her blow her nose clean. Again, we applauded all of her efforts. The next step was to play a game and ask if she could make the water come out of the other nostril. Over a short period, Brianna became an expert at independent washing.

Four-year-old Sophie's speech development was delayed because of recurrent ear problems caused by allergies. Sophie slowly learned to use a nasal wash much like Brianna. Only one year later, Sophie's parents report that when she wakes up with a stuffy nose she'll ask to wash. Then she steps up to the sink, washes her nose completely on her own, blows, grunts like an old man and walks away saying "Now that feels good. I can breathe."

Never introduce a child to nose washing by doing it to them. Children want to be empowered, not controlled. This was made very clear to me when I saw my own two-year-old grandson resisting his parents' efforts to wash his nose. So instead of bringing out the bottle and trying to chase him down, I spent time with him watching videos of other children washing, time playing with the bottle as a squirty toy, and talking about how good a clean nose feels. We agreed: he could run faster and wouldn't need to take medicine so much if he had a clean nose. Before his parents knew it, Eliot was washing his nose like a pro - all on his own, happy and proud to be in control.

The overall approach to teach a child how to wash must be geared towards the child's developmental age as well as his or her past experiences. One slow step at a time, no forcing allowed. Only gentle encouragement, demonstrations and lots of positives for any success at all.

How to Teach
Your Two to Three-Year-Old Toddler to Wash

 It can be difficult to get toddlers to do anything they think is suspect, so you may have a challenge ahead of you. But the effort is worth it. My best advice is to proceed slowly, be resolved to succeed, and always remember that children learn best by playing, doing and imitating what you do. Teaching a toddler to wash her nose is much like the way you teach a two-year-old to brush her teeth: one step at a time, no forcing, no pressure, no trauma - only fun and rewards and repeated demonstrations of good technique. You improve the technique one step at a time. Begin by feeling comfortable washing your own nose, so that your child will see and feel your comfort level.

Next, allow plenty of bathtub play involving a nasal wash bottle, allowing your child to get comfortable holding and squirting the bottle. Play "squirty" games with your child. Suggest, "Let's wash her tummy - squirt! Let's wash her ears - squirt! Wash her knees - squirt! Wash her nose - squirt!" Make this game a nightly routine.

Once comfortable, add your child's face parts to your squirty games as you continue to squirt the cheeks, lips, outer nose - don't forget to giggle and laugh with your child, and be sure to avoid the eyes. Be very matter-of-fact and make it a natural part of the game. Say "This is fun!" Do not say, "See, that doesn't hurt!"

After your child is comfortable having water in her face, she may want to wipe it off with a wash cloth each time she is squirted, and that's okay too. It is time to start washing the inside of her nose. Begin with a mild saline solution and a full bottle of warm water. The solution temperature should be the same as the bath water temperature. Keep playing the same games - squirt the baby doll, squirt your child's belly button, ears, etc. Then say, "Let's wash inside your nose a little, too," and ask her to place the tip near her nose and squeeze. She may need a bit of guidance with your hand to make sure the bottle is held correctly but allow her to have all the control. Don't squeeze the bottle for her. Move right on and say, "Let's wash your big toe -squirt!" Giggle! "Let's wash your belly button -squirt!" Giggle! "Let's wash your OTHER nose - squirt!" Giggle!

The idea is to keep moving, keep your child distracted and keep it a game. If your child backs away, go back to the point of comfort in the squirty games for several days. Once she is calm and playful, begin advancing the process again, but slower. Allow your child to have control by letting her squirt you a lot more. Eventually move back to her ears, nose, forehead, etc. Realize that for naturally fearful children this process may take weeks of "two steps forward, one step back" progress. Do not become discouraged, but remain upbeat. It is important to allow game-playing, rewards, clapping and positive reinforcement to rule your behavior. Allow your child as much autonomy as possible - which may be choosing which doll, the color towel to dry off with, or the sticker she is going to put on her chart - because this will decrease the struggles you encounter. It may take some trial and error on your part - like much of parenting.

If you invite your toddler to watch you wash daily, it can become a routine.

A Dad's Success Story with His Three-Year-Old

66 *I have been washing for about a year and am still enjoying how clean my sinuses feel after the shower. I do have one story to share where I ended up using the nose wash with my three-year-old daughter. She was playing with play-dough one afternoon and she must have put a small piece in her nose. I tried everything I could think of to get it out and was getting worried that she might inhale too hard and get it really stuck. So I decided to rinse her nostrils out. Well, after a few moments of the fluid sitting in her nose the piece just fell out. I was so happy that I had that nose wash bottle to get that piece out of her nose.* **99**

Charles L., Ledgewood, New Jersey

How to Teach
Your Four to Six-Year-Old to Wash

"I can do it myself!" Four to six years is certainly the "I can do it myself" age - if only they could! Begin by allowing your child plenty of play time in the tub with the nasal wash bottle to acquire a familiarity with it. It is important to keep in mind that children this age also learn by playing, by exploring and by doing.

Children this age like to have an assigned task. Explain why it is important to get the old, thick, crusty mucus out of their nose. Try a creative, simplistic approach such as the nose being like a cave, with big booger rocks blocking the entrance. Calling the bottle a "booger blaster" adds a little element of excitement and may help your child envision just what his task involves.

Always give your child many opportunities to watch you wash your nose. Any comments from you regarding, "Boy, that feels good. Now I can breathe," communicates that what you are requesting is a habit you yourself enjoy. A sticker chart encourages compliance with the daily task and rewards your child's efforts with no nagging on your part. Make a target out of a plastic plate, with circles marked off in permanent marker, and attach it to the shower wall. Begin by having your child practice aiming the squirt bottle and hitting a bull's eye on the target during bath time each evening for a week or so to prove his aim is good enough to take on the task of nose washing by himself. This will put him into a competitive, self-empowered mood.

Once your child is comfortable, make up an isotonic salt solution and have him gently squirt the solution inside his nose, with lots of praise, whooping, clapping and sideline cheering. Immediately have him climb out of the tub and put his sticker on his reward chart. It is vitally important to remember that children this age have a very short attention span and need instant feedback and reward. You will have to be consistent in your effort to train him to be consistent in his. Nose washing can take place in the bath, the kitchen sink, or even outdoors. Experiment with your child. Play with the bottle. Make a game out of it.

How to Teach
Your Seven to Nine-Year-Old to Wash

 This section assumes that your child has been exposed to some water play, likes a little adventure, and is not afraid to put her face in the water. Encouraging your child to "face up" into the shower may also take away the notion that it is somehow harmful to get water in our faces, ears, eyes or nose. Blowing bubbles with the mouth or even the nose in the clean bath water, or encouraging the shower water to fall directly onto the face may help take away any fear of water in the face.

Then it is time to get down to business. Kids at this age are usually very interested in bodily functions, so they're fascinated at the idea that mucus which is allowed to stand inside their nose and sinuses transforms into nasty stuff that needs to be cleaned out. Demonstrate your technique to reassure your child that this squirt into their nose will come back out.

While being gently firm about the necessity of this activity, turn it into a game. They can understand the idea of their nose and sinuses being like a cave. Inside, it is dark and warm, with moisture dripping off the walls. The moisture collects on the floor and hardens, forming "snot-rocks," or pools of "booger juice." If allowed to continue, this nasty stuff can clog up their cave. If they want the "air carriers" to be allowed through, they must wash out the nasty stuff and keep the passages clean of snot-rocks. Girls this age may like a game of a princess, pony or a benevolent being living in the back of a cave which needs to be kept clean for access to the world beyond. Kids this age have great imaginations. If allowed to make up their own story about their cave, and the reason they must sweep it clean with a water hose every day, you will find they are much more compliant, because the story almost becomes real for them. Positive reinforcement for such compliance works better than nagging about non-compliance. Take a deep breath, both of you will survive!

The best medicine often makes good sense. Just keep your nose clean.

Blow, Blow, Blow Your Nose
Gently Now, Don't Scream

 Teaching your toddler or preschooler how to blow his nose may have developed into your greatest challenge as a parent thus far! We all get tired of seeing goopy-nosed little ones running around, and wish there was an easy way to teach them to just blow all that junk out, with or without our help.

Remember that while breathing in and out is a natural, instinctive ability, blowing in and out - either through the mouth or the nose - is a learned behavior. It is also a rather abstract idea, and while young children are good at concrete concepts, most of them flounder when it comes to abstract thinking. So if your kid gets this quickly, consider him or her a genius!

First, practice blowing air through the mouth. Buy a large bottle of bubbles with a wand and teach your child to blow bubbles. Emphasize gentle pursing of the lips as well as puffing the air as you enjoy watching the bubbles form.

Now practice blowing air through the nose and not the mouth. Start with "Blow the Hankie." Get a tissue. Have your child take a deep breath and clamp her teeth together. Gently hold your index finger up and down across her lips as though you are telling her to shush. Hold the tissue about an inch from her face and see if she can move it by blowing the air from her nose. If she does, SHE WINS! It may help to have her gently close off one nostril and blow through just one side at a time. This seems to help some children feel the air move through their nose while keeping their mouth closed, which is the key - and the hardest concept for children to grasp.

Be prepared to provide lots of clapping and cheering and encouragement during these games, as well as reminders about keeping lips sealed shut, breathing in and out through the nose only, etc. Only give positives for any attempt. No negatives, ever! With practice, all children will learn if the task is a fun game and not a chore.

What If Your Preschool Child Is Scared of Water?

 I have often heard a mother say, "My child is terrified of water and you want me to put water in his nose?"

First we must understand that survival is a basic instinct, so it is not just oppositional behavior that makes a child scream at the perception that he may drown.

Begin by allowing your child to stand on the bath mat in a couple of inches of water, bathing his toys and toes slowly and gently. You may want to run warm water into the tub and turn off the water before you even take him in the bathroom. The loud sound of water running can be frightening to some sensitive children.

Assure him that from now on he may just stand in the tub while you wipe him down with a wet cloth. That's all. Give him control and he will amaze you.

Put some tub toys to float in the water. Over a matter of weeks, slowly raise the depth of the water to his mid-shin. If you make no threats, odds are he will begin to play with the floating toys, eventually sitting in the water.

Slowly now, when washing him, begin to drizzle a bit of water on his skin playfully, from the tip of the washcloth. Over the week ahead, drizzle a bit more. The idea is to slowly desensitize him until he is used to having water touching him, splashing on him, eventually in his face, without setting off a panic attack.

Once you have your child sitting in the shallow water at play, don't say anything about it. Treat it as a non-event. Never, never say, "See, there is nothing to be afraid of." That simply reminds the child of his fear, and makes him begin to worry again that maybe he was right. If you can manage to turn this around and teach him how to wash in general, he will eventually learn to wash his nose. Once a child has developed a fearful response, it will take many safe, pleasurable experiences to replace those original memories, so patience is of the essence.

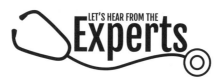

Irrigation, not Operation

Good results with nasal irrigation are not limited to adults. Many children can benefit from nasal washing as well. Because of the limited treatment options to control nasal congestion, runny nose, and cough in children younger than twelve, washing becomes even more important in this age group. The FDA in October 2008 recommended that over-the-counter cold medication not be used in children under four years of age. Additionally, the agency cautioned that these drugs may not be safe in children from two to twelve years old. To control symptoms, parents have been encouraged to return to simpler, more natural remedies, including nasal saline drops for infants and washing for older children. Many of the children have had numerous ear infections but always seem to have a runny nose and chronic congestion. When properly instructed by their doctors and coached by their parents, nose washing can successfully be used to treat nasal symptoms in children and to help decrease colds, sore throats, and ear infections.

Washing helps clear nasal secretions that can lead to chronic sniffling. I have often thought that if kids could just blow their nose they could alleviate many of their upper respiratory and ear complaints. Washing is able to help clear young noses.

Chronic sniffling can lead to negative pressure in the middle ear. This negative pressure can pull tissue fluid into the middle ear causing pain and decreased hearing. Have you have ever been on airplane and not been able to clear your ears? That's the type of discomfort a child may feel when the pressure hits. No wonder they can be cranky.

In the case of "Jamie," this four-year-old was working on getting his second set of ear tubes. He got his first set of tubes when he was eleven months old. They stayed in for two and a half years. Well, that's how long he went before having another infection. Before the ear surgery there were lots of sleepless nights and lots of trips to the doctor's office. The parents were concerned the cycle may be repeating itself again. Increasingly, Jamie was complaining about earaches. The parents were not sure if he had selective hearing loss or if his hearing may actually have been getting worse.

Even though the family was quick to seek consultation with an ENT (Ear, nose, and throat specialist) after having an initial good experience with ear tubes, they were hesitant to have surgery again. They were spending more time at the lake and wanted Jamie to start swimming lessons. They were concerned about scarring in his eardrums.

Except for some allergies, Jamie was a healthy young boy. He just seemed to always have a runny nose. Try as they might, his parents were unable to teach him to blow his nose. Jamie was too busy "doing boy stuff" to care; a long sniff of his nose or wipe of his nose with his hand was fine with him. When his allergies got bad the family relied on oral antihistamines.

On exam, Jamie seemed to be a happy, healthy child. His nose was somewhat congested with a mild increase in drainage. In general, he had a good nasal airway, mostly breathing through his nose. His tonsils were not particularly enlarged.

His ears, however, were full of fluid. The retracted nature of the ear drum and the light tan color of the fluid suggested to me that he had a thick mucus effusion resulting in a blockage-type hearing loss (conductive loss) usually corrected by treating the effusion. A hearing test confirmed that he had a 25db conductive hearing loss. I explained to the parents that this was comparable to walking around with fingers in your ears.

Usually when there is hearing loss, I tend to be more aggressive in suggesting tubes. Going into the summer months, with his desire to swim and considering his history of poorly controlled nasal symptoms, I felt it was important to give him a chance at conservative management. I strongly felt that clearing up his nose would be his best chance of avoiding surgery. Drying up his nose seemed like an impossible dream to his mother, who had long complained about the constant drip.

After reviewing the options with the family, I began to suggest nasal washing. I explained how the Nasopure system was designed with the young nose in mind. I explained the steps to success that others had followed, including parental encouragement and demonstration. Kids who see the parents washing their nose are more likely to try it. It also helps to allow the child to play with the irrigation bottle during bath time, introducing nasal washing to him over time.

Four weeks later at his follow up visit, I was happy to hear that Jamie had mastered the irrigation technique and mom was happy that his nose was clean. Jamie was actually asking for the irrigation because he liked having a clean nose too.

He still had fluid in his ears, but now the retraction of the eardrum was much less and there were a few air bubbles in the middle ear. The return of air to the middle ear was a certain sign we were on the right track. Over the next few weeks he was able to clear his ears and successfully avoid surgery.

Nasal washing may not always be practical in children younger than two. But it can almost always be tried in older children to either prevent surgery or to avoid the need for a second and third set of ear tubes.

Kelvin Walls, MD
Otolaryngologist (aka ENT; Ears, Nose, Throat--Head and Neck Surgeon)
Lees Summit, Missouri

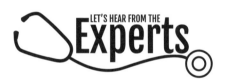

LET'S HEAR FROM THE
Experts

These are the x-ray images of a 35-month old boy who had almost continuous purulent rhinorrhea (thick runny nose) and cough over a two year period. He attends a preschool with 19 other children. He frequently experienced fevers, requiring many courses of antibiotics, and typically had relapses within the first six days off antibiotics. This pattern continued despite having an adenoidectomy (removal of the adenoids) four months earlier.

The view on the left shows cloudy maxillary (below the eyes) and ethmoid (between the eyes) sinuses, with only a small amount of air in the left maxillary sinus (arrow).

A dose of 23-valent pneumococcal vaccine was given, and twice-daily hypertonic buffered nasal saline irrigation prescribed. (Yes, a 35-month-old child did have twice daily nasal washes!)

He returned 21 days later with no interim flare, six weeks since his last antibiotics, having only mild residual rhinorrhea and occasional cough. An x-ray (right), showed marked clearing of both maxillary sinuses. The ethmoid sinuses remain opacified but improved.

During the interim he had received every dose of the prescribed nasal saline irrigation, with no other medications. Responses to the pneumococcal vaccine were excellent.

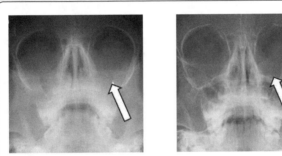

The view on the left shows cloudy maxillary (below the eyes) and ethmoid (between the eyes) sinuses prior to nasal irrigation.

The x-ray on the right, taken 3 weeks after daily nasal washing shows marked clearing (less cloudy) of both maxillary sinuses. The ethmoids remained opacified but improved.

Michael Cooperstock, MD, MPH
Pediatric Infectious Disease
University of Missouri, Columbia, Medical Center

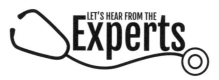

Rinsing Away Kids' Allergies

Hypertonic nasal saline irrigation is something that I recommend quite often to my patients. People of all ages benefit from the decongesting, bacteriostatic action that hypertonic saline provides. Dr. Hana has done something quite unique with her product. Not only does she provide the ingredients and means to do the saline wash, she has clear, concise directions for how to effectively get the job done. This is especially an issue when dealing with children. Her written directions for different age groups and video of a four-year-old washing her nose so easily are fabulous resources for patients (and parents) to utilize.

Laurie Fowler, MD
Fowler Allergy Clinic
Columbia, Missouri

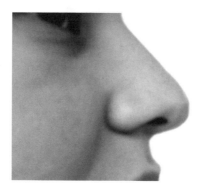

Chapter 9

Just for Women

Pregnancy and Hormones

 At least twenty to thirty percent of pregnant women suffer from Pregnancy Induced Rhinitis (PIR), a condition that causes nasal congestion and other symptoms that include sneezing, nasal itching, persistent coughing, snoring, fatigue, and even headaches. Breathing can be so uncomfortable it interferes with sleep, forcing a woman to continually breathe out of her mouth. Congestion and fatigue can lead to ear and sinus infections, further complicating the situation. This leads desperate pregnant women to try anything to help them breathe and feel better, but their options are limited.

True PIR goes away within two weeks after delivering the baby. This makes us think the cause may be related to placental growth hormone. Allergies to dust mites have also been implicated as a risk factor for PIR, and we know that if a woman smokes cigarettes, her risk of developing PIR increases to almost 70%.

Initially it may be difficult to tell the difference between PIR and allergies or sinus infections. Over-the-counter and prescription medications to treat severe congestion are not without risks during pregnancy, and in reality may not be effective or even needed.

Symptoms of Pregnancy-Induced Rhinitis

- Nasal congestion
- Sneezing
- Coughing
- Runny nose
- Facial pressure
- Sinus congestion
- Headaches

Many women's first thought for relief might be to use a decongestant pill such as pseudoephedrine (Sudafed), but the effects of decongestants on a developing fetus have not yet been adequately studied. Since PIR is not an allergic reaction, antihistamines may not help, instead bringing unwanted side effects that further dry the nasal passages. Topical decongestants in the form of nasal sprays may give temporary relief, but they quickly become habit-forming, leading to the condition known as Rhinitis Medicamentosa (see pg. XX). Topical steroid sprays have not been shown to help open the nose and the body absorbs some of the steroids, giving the fetus a dose that may not be healthy.

So what *does* work? And what *is* safe to use during pregnancy?

Conservative management is not only the safest route to take when it comes to PIR, but it has also been shown to be the most effective. Elevate the head of the bed 35-40 degrees to reduce night-time congestion and pressure. Non-impact, moderate exercise decreases nasal congestion and rhinitis symptoms. Drinking plenty of fluids, especially those without caffeine, can help, as can taking a steaming hot shower. In severe cases, CPAP (Continuous Positive Airway Pressure) while sleeping has been used with good results. Some women have even used mechanical nasal dilators to get relief.

But the safest, easiest, and often the most effective treatment for PIR has been proven to be nasal washes with hypertonic saline solution. Warm saline washing soothes irritated tissue, improves the sense of smell, liquefies sticky thick mucus, and aids in tissue repair. If the solution is hypertonic (saltier than the body), it acts as a natural decongestant without the side effects of pills or sprays. And it can be used as often as necessary; there is no problem with washing four or five times a day if that is what keeps the nose open and breathing comfortably.

Pregnancy is a precious time in a woman's life, and if a problem like PIR develops, it can be difficult to enjoy. If you can't breathe, it is difficult to get enough sleep, to eat well, to exercise and otherwise prepare for the arrival of a new baby. And let's face it, there are few smells sweeter than that of a newborn baby. If PIR takes two weeks to resolve after the baby is born, just think - a new mother loses that aspect of those precious days of bonding. Our sense of smell is so important, to say nothing of being able to breathe! If nose washing can allow a mother to fully appreciate her baby, it's a solution that can't be ignored.

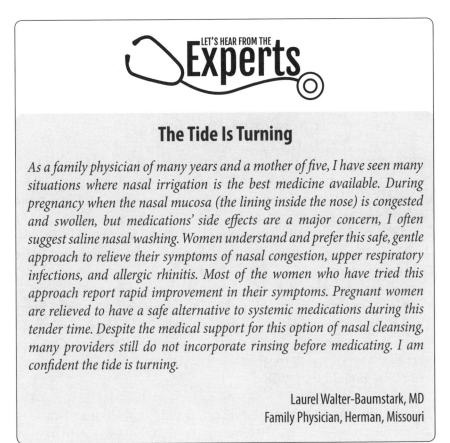

LET'S HEAR FROM THE Experts

The Tide Is Turning

As a family physician of many years and a mother of five, I have seen many situations where nasal irrigation is the best medicine available. During pregnancy when the nasal mucosa (the lining inside the nose) is congested and swollen, but medications' side effects are a major concern, I often suggest saline nasal washing. Women understand and prefer this safe, gentle approach to relieve their symptoms of nasal congestion, upper respiratory infections, and allergic rhinitis. Most of the women who have tried this approach report rapid improvement in their symptoms. Pregnant women are relieved to have a safe alternative to systemic medications during this tender time. Despite the medical support for this option of nasal cleansing, many providers still do not incorporate rinsing before medicating. I am confident the tide is turning.

Laurel Walter-Baumstark, MD
Family Physician, Herman, Missouri

Pregnant and Healthy

···

66 *I am 26 weeks pregnant with our first child, a son! And I believe that using nasal washing every day has helped me keep common colds at bay. The cold that I am currently getting over now did not get very bad at all. When I started to feel sick I started washing morning and night; that, I believe, helped me from feeling like I'd been hit by a truck. I didn't need or want to take medicine to feel better!* **99**

Janis M., Springfield, Illinois

···

Women and Heart Disease:
Is Air Pollution a Factor?

 In 2007, the New England Journal of Medicine published a study involving almost 66,000 postmenopausal women. Researchers examined the association of cardiovascular events (heart problems) with long-term exposure to tiny particulate matter. They found a strong correlation, showing that exposure to fine grit in polluted air boosts the risk of heart disease in women.

It has long been known that air pollution contributes to lung and heart disease, with women perhaps more susceptible than men. This study looked at deaths as well as heart attacks, coronary disease, strokes and clogged arteries. These problems were 24% more likely with every ten-unit rise in pollution particles.

The tiny unit particles (vehicle exhaust, factory dust, soot and various chemicals) are so small that 30 bits equal the width of a strand of human hair. This is an example of a situation where nasal irrigation can remove these particles from the nose before they can enter the lungs and cause long-term damage. We can lower the pollution level in our nose while we work on lowering the pollution level in our communities.

Chapter 10

The Seasoned Schnozz

 Much like the rest of the body, the nose experiences change as we mature. We may become wiser, but some parts do not work as well as when we were younger. With age, there is an increased likelihood of certain nasal ailments, including increased airflow resistance: we become more congested as we age. Mature patients frequently experience an uncomfortable dry nose and recurrent crusting.

There is a natural physiological phenomenon of alternating congestion and decongestion of the nasal airways. Most people are never aware of these fluctuations. Nasal challenges in the seasoned nose are a consequence of lower intranasal air temperature and lower humidity, combined with relatively enlarged nasal cavities. This enlargement is due to involution - a shrinking away or atrophy of the nasal membranes *(mucosa)*.

We need to be mindful that taking additional medications is not a wise idea, especially for more mature patients. Moisturizing and cleansing the nasal cavity can significantly improve quality of life and further increase the enjoyment of stopping to smell the roses.

Points to remember for the seasoned nose:
- ✓ Mucus is thicker and stickier due to hormonal changes.
- ✓ Medications can have negative results on mucus consistency.
- ✓ There may be a decreased ability to detect odors.
- ✓ Tissues shrink with age.
- ✓ Moisture becomes more difficult to maintain.
- ✓ Sense of smell and taste are connected. As you age you have fewer taste buds, so the nose becomes more important to compensate for that loss.

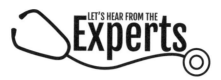

Finally, Relief!

Mary is a middle-aged woman who has suffered with sinus problems her whole adult life. When her complaints of congestion, headaches, nasal drainage, and facial pressure became severe enough she turned to over-the-counter medication, which she had used without success. When she got tired of being sick and missing work she would go to her doctor.

Through the years she has seen primary care physicians and specialists to help her with her sinus symptoms. She has been on many rounds of antibiotics, nasal steroid sprays and antihistamines, at times responding to treatment only to have a recurrence of her symptoms. It was not uncommon for her to have four to five sinus infections per year. In addition to her sinus complaints, which included facial pressure / pain and popping in her ears, she also complained of postnasal drainage that made her sick, starting with a sore throat then getting down into her chest, making her cough and leading to bronchitis. Not long after the coughing started she would lose her voice. Then she would be unable to work. In fact, it was the bronchitis, the coughing, the lack of sleep and the inability to work that usually drove her to the doctor.

I saw her after she had persistent symptoms even though she had followed her prescribed treatment. She was very frustrated and was becoming increasingly concerned about the fact the she was, as she put it, "living on antibiotics." CT scan evaluation of her sinuses confirmed sinus disease. Because she was afraid of losing her job she was reluctant to proceed with surgery. In addition to her current sinus medications, I started her on a regimen of hypertonic saline irrigation.

Even though she was in an "I will try anything" mode, she was skeptical about nasal irrigation. She made it clear to me that she didn't like putting anything in her nose. After an explanation of the technique she agreed to try it.

At follow-up she was overwhelmed with how well it had worked. For the first time she was "clear!" She was able to breathe through her nose. The drainage had stopped for the first time in a long time. The headaches were gone and she was resting better. Her voice was back to normal and her throat didn't feel irritated all the time.

On long-term follow-up, she still hasn't scheduled that sinus surgery. Oh, she still gets sinus infections; they just don't control her life any more. The mild symptoms she now has are manageable. It doesn't get "down into her chest." Her sinus infection and colds are much less frequent. And when she does get one, it does not last nearly as long. She is not missing nearly as much work.

Kelvin Walls, MD
Otolaryngologist (ENT; Ears, Nose, Throat--Head and Neck Surgeon)
Lees Summit, Missouri

LET'S HEAR FROM THE
Experts

Worth Waiting For

My introduction to the idea of nasal irrigation came many years ago when patients started telling me about the "neti pot" - an ancient ceramic device that holds a saline solution and has a spout that is inserted into each nostril and tipped up to pour the liquid into the nose and out the mouth or other nostril. I looked into this method and even bought a neti pot for my own use. I found the cleansing outcome very helpful, but the process seemed awkward and difficult to master. Then a few years ago I heard about the Nasopure product. The concept of nasal irrigation to cleanse the nasal passages is the same, but the actual process of irrigation using this device is so much simpler than the neti pot.

I have many patients who have found benefit from this system. Anyone with recurrent sinus problems, allergy symptoms involving the nose and throat, recurrent ear or Eustachian tube issues benefits from daily nasal irrigation with a mild saline solution.

One recent example is Teri, a 40-year-old woman with recurrent sinus infections repeatedly treated with antibiotics. Once she began regular saline nasal irrigations, she noticed immediate improvement. She has needed no antibiotics now for several years! She and I are very grateful for this most useful, health-saving technique!

Julia, another middle-aged woman, was plagued every spring and summer with seasonal allergies. She experienced sneezing, coughing, itchy eyes and runny nose. Her tolerance for oral allergy medications was not good - they all made her sleepy. Once she started saline irrigations regularly, her allergy symptoms abated almost completely. She, too, is a believer in the very beneficial health effects of nasal washing.

My regular recommendation now to all patients who have any chronic nasal, sinus or other upper respiratory symptoms is to use saline irrigation on a regular basis - daily for maintenance of good health, and twice a day if they are feeling more congested or beginning to get allergy symptoms or a stuffy nose. It makes so much sense to wash out the part of our body that must filter all the microscopic particles in the air we breathe every minute of every day. We wash our skin, our hair and our teeth regularly - now we can also wash our nasal passages!

Jane Murray, MD
Family Physician, Sastun Center
Overland Park, Kansas

Dad Learns To Wash

❝ *My 87-year-old dad is flying to England and uses his nasal wash system every day. In addition to his constant cough for 30 years that he finally got rid of two years ago when I took a nasal wash device to him, just recently he has completely gotten rid of his psoriasis. In retrospect, I think the constant inflammatory process in his throat drained his body of anti-inflammatory nutrients and so one malady leads to the next and the next. By curing his sinus and throat problems, his skin had a chance to heal completely. If my dad could learn to use a nasal wash system effectively, I think just about anyone who is fairly spry could learn to do it. It certainly has made a great improvement for my dad. Whether or not the psoriasis stopped because of nasal washing is hard to prove but getting rid of a difficult problem, like a chronic throat-choking cough, can free the immune system to heal other parts of the body.* **❞**

Marilyn W, St Louis, Missouri

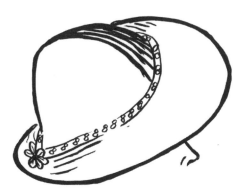

Chapter 11

When Your Defense Is Down

 The following is a compilation of my clinical experiences and the opinions of some of my colleagues. The conditions noted are not intended to be 100% inclusive of what can go wrong when our defenses are down, but rather are examples of common conditions related to the nose.

Viral Infections

The Common Cold and That Dreaded Flu Virus

First, a few notes regarding the differences between colds and influenza. The Centers for Disease Control and Prevention (CDC) recognizes that most folks do not really understand the difference between these two viral illnesses, yet the difference can be deadly.

Influenza, commonly called "the flu," is caused by the *influenza virus*. This is a specific respiratory virus quite different than the cold virus. The entire respiratory tract, including the nose, throat and lungs, becomes infected. The illness is severe and can be life threatening; children, the elderly and those who have underlying medical conditions are at greatest risk for complications.

Full-blown symptoms of the flu often develop suddenly. "I was fine before lunch, and then I suddenly felt really ill by two pm. It was like I was hit by a Mack truck." Symptoms include fever, headache, extreme tiredness, dry cough, sore throat, runny or stuffy nose, and significant muscle aches. Children can also have nausea, vomiting, and diarrhea.

The nose is the primary invasion route for respiratory viruses, so here is where its job of filtering is so vitally important. Both influenza and cold viruses are spread mainly through respiratory droplets - spread by coughs and sneezes from infected people. A typical sneeze can propel up to one hundred thousand droplets through the air. The droplets can survive anywhere from a few seconds up to forty-eight hours, so it is possible to be exposed by touching a surface that was sneezed on or touched by infected hands earlier in the day.

The clinical difference between the flu and a cold is this: the flu symptoms and possible complications are much worse than the common cold. The fever, body aches, extreme tiredness, and dry cough of the flu are more intense. Colds usually do not develop into pneumonia, secondary bacterial infections, or require hospitalization.

A clear distinction I see as a medical provider between a common cold and the flu is this: a person with a cold will walk normally into the clinic, complain miserably about their symptoms, but will admit that only their head and neck are affected. They may complain of a cough and tightness in their chest, but they will not be incapacitated. Someone with influenza appears quite ill, is barely able to climb onto the exam table, and the entire body is affected - every muscle feeling sore, tired and toxic. Most patients with influenza are unable to leave their house and wait for several days before seeing a doctor, saying, "I was too sick to come in."

So how serious is the influenza virus? Based on the best data we can access, each year between 5% and 20% of the U.S. population will get the flu. About 200,000 will be hospitalized with complications and each year, anywhere from 3,000 to 49,000 will die from flu-related complications. These complications include ear infections, sinus infections, bronchitis and pneumonia - with pneumonia being the most deadly, especially to those who are very young or very old.

So you can see how important it is to take aggressive measures to prevent infection in the first place!

Comparison Between the Common Cold and the Influenza Virus

	COLD	INFLUENZA
Onset	Gradual Onset 1-3 Days	Sudden Onset 3-6 Hours
Fever	Rare, Low Grade	Yes, High Grade
Chills	Uncommon	Common
Cough	Mild, Post Nasal Drip	Yes
Body Aches	None - Slight	Severe Muscle Aches
Fatigue	None - Mild	Moderate - Severe
Appetite	Normal - Mild Decrease	Decreased - Absent
Nose	Stuffy, Drippy, Sneezy	Slightly Stuffy
Headache	Uncommon	Common

Yearly flu vaccines are developed just for this purpose: prevention of serious influenza infections. But the flu virus mutates on a regular basis, so the flu that was a problem last year may not be the one to avoid this year. These mutations also mean that our own immune systems cannot completely protect us from year to year based on past experience. To account for this yearly change in viral form, each year the developers of the flu vaccine make an educated guess when they create the next year's vaccine and most of the time they get it right. But sometimes the virus fools everyone and the vaccine is not as effective as hoped.

Remembering that most viruses enter through the nose reminds us that this is where the function of the nose as a filter is extremely important. Keeping that filter in good working order is essential during cold and flu season, and hypertonic washing is always effective, no matter how often viruses change their shape or form. Washing out viral particles before they have a chance to invade the mucosa is powerful prevention.

Bottom line: Getting an annual flu shot, practicing good public hygiene habits, and washing your nasal filter regularly can give you the best protection from both the influenza and the common cold virus.

The Common Cold

 Most adults have two to four colds a year and normal children can have up to nine per year. Despite the name, colds are not caused by winter weather, cold temperatures or even an uncovered head or neck. Humans spread the virus, especially as we spend more time indoors during the holidays, sharing the air we breathe. Do you think it is a coincidence that the return from holiday travels always seems to bring on colds? I believe that with age and exposure, one develops immunity to familiar viruses, but when we travel to another part of the country and share new germs, within three to seven days a new cold virus can be spreading through your home. Once someone sneezes or coughs, the viral droplets can travel several feet and land onto another's mouth, nose or hard surface just to be relocated by a human hand. Air travel is a notorious example of this.

Rhinovirus, the most frequent cause of the common cold, has more than 100 different varieties. Developing immunity to one type does nothing to keep the others from attacking and ruining your week.

Two studies found that nose washing can take a lot of the misery out of the common cold. Consistently, over 20 years, I have confirmed this to be true in my patients.

In the fall of 1998, Dr. Richard Ravizza, MD at Pennsylvania State University presented his findings to the 50th Scientific Assembly of the American Academy of Family Physicians. In this study, 294 college students were divided into three subgroups. One subgroup performed daily nasal irrigation, one took a daily placebo pill, and the third group was left untreated. All participants were asked to keep a cold symptoms diary. The study found that students who used the daily saline rinse experienced a significant reduction in the number of colds contracted compared with non-users. On average, those engaging in nasal irrigation had fewer colds over the study period compared with the placebo or untreated groups.

A study published in the January 2008 issue of Archives of *Otolaryngology* found that a saline nasal wash solution improves nasal symptoms and may help prevent the recurrence of respiratory infections when used by children with the common cold. The researchers studied the cold and flu symptoms, consumption of medication, complications, days off school as well as the number of illness days during follow up visits. The patients in the saline group showed significantly lower scores in sore throat, cough, nasal obstruction, and secretion. By the third follow-up visit, significantly fewer children in the saline group as compared to the control group were using fever reducing medications (9% vs. 33%), nasal decongestants (5% vs. 47%), mucolytics (10% vs. 37%), and systemic antibiotics and antiviral medications (6% vs. 21%). During the same period children in the saline group also reported significantly fewer illness days (31% vs. 75%), school absences (17% vs. 35%), and complications (8% vs. 32%). The nasal wash was well tolerated.

This study was released as other researchers were reporting that non-prescription cough medicines do not help children with colds and might even cause harm. Another study suggested that these cold medications don't help adults much, either.

In my experience with patients there isn't much mystery. Colds, typically lasting seven to ten days, are spread by respiratory *(aerosol)* droplets. If one sneezes or coughs, these droplets travel approximately six feet, and are inhaled by someone in the room or sharing the same air. Saline washes work by removing inflammatory compounds and by creating a favorable environment for cilia to sweep away mucus and viral particles.

Dr. Hana's
CLINICAL ●PEARLS

Stay Moistened, Stay Hydrated, Stay Warm and Rested.

Everyone has some advice on treating a cold, so I want to share mine.

There are three key supportive measures, which can help you while avoiding secondary bacterial infections.

- ✓ STAY HYDRATED: Maintain adequate fluids, both inside and out. A guide for what is adequate for your internal needs is the number of times you need to empty your bladder - it should be at least four times each day. Appropriate fluid sources include soups, water, and fruits, but not caffeine.
- ✓ STAY MOISTENED: To keep the mucus loose, take long warm baths or showers often and maintain the humidity in the air you breathe. Wash the nasal cavity clean of infected mucus.
- ✓ STAY WARM AND RESTED: Sleep often, sleep well.

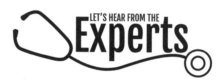

Large influenza epidemics occur almost every winter. About 1/3 of the population typically becomes infected. It is the worst of the common respiratory viruses, causing an average of about 200,000 hospitalizations and 34,000 deaths each year. Many of the hospitalizations occur in infants, a few of whom die. Children with sinus problems or frequent ear infections are almost sure to have a relapse if they develop influenza. This can be minimized or prevented with influenza shots for the whole family each October. In children, the new live, attenuated nasal influenza vaccine works even better. It is a more natural way to immunize, and lasts longer than the injectable vaccine, even into the following year. The protection is also somewhat stronger. Finally, the protection is also broader, working well when epidemic strains "drift" away from the protectiveness of injectable vaccine, a problem which happens to some extent in most years.

Michael Cooperstock, MD, MPH
Pediatric Infectious Disease
University of Missouri, Columbia, Medical Center

Reminders When You Have a Cold

✓ Start self-care measures at the very first hint of a cold's onset.
✓ Don't rub your eyes.
✓ Cold viruses love eyes and noses but rarely leap mouth to mouth.
✓ Keep the mucus flowing out.
✓ Stay hydrated.
✓ Skip antihistamines, which can dry nasal membranes and slow the mucus flow.
✓ Decongestants can help ease stuffiness because they shrink swollen tissue inside the noses. But remember, nasal decongestant sprays can worsen congestion if used for more than two or three days (see Chapter 3 Rhinitis Medicamentosa).
✓ Humidity helps reduce congestion.
✓ Soups (yes, chicken soup) and most warm fluids are helpful. The warmth helps loosen the mucus; the nutrients are good for you.
✓ Be patient. Whether you treat the cold at home, or go to the doctor, a typical cold will still last about seven to ten days.
✓ Most treatments address only the cold symptoms, not the underlying infection.
✓ Avoid Eskimo kisses and other intimate contact with those you love
✓ And YES, wash your nose!

Breathing!

66 *It felt amazing at first because I forgot what it was like to breathe through my nose. I now have less congestion and it prevents chest colds from starting.* 99

David C., College student in Texas

Keep the System Clean

66 *In my opinion, preventing colds - and a variety of other sicknesses as well - is as simple as good hygiene. We all know that washing our hands is important, but I noticed a big difference when I took the next step: washing my nose. We breathe in thousands of gallons of air every day, along with dirt, irritating chemicals, germs, viruses and whatever else the air bears. Once I got in the habit of rinsing my nose out with warm saline once a day and saw all the icky stuff that rinsing brought out, I hated to miss even a single day.* 99

Nick Kasoff, Radio DJ, St. Louis, Missouri

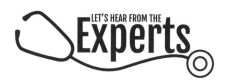

Day care can provide developmentally important experiences for preschoolers while allowing parents to pursue careers. It also exposes youngsters to a great many infections. The larger the center, the greater the risk. Once the daycare group increases beyond more than about six children, the risk of infections increases dramatically. Children in large day care centers have more infections of almost every kind, and require antibiotics more often for bacterial infections that are more likely to be resistant to antimicrobials.

Michael Cooperstock, MD, MPH
Pediatric Infectious Disease
University of Missouri, Columbia, Medical Center

Avoiding the Common Cold

❝ *While on a trip in November, I noticed stuffiness and some post nasal drainage beginning, and with just one washing that disappeared. Since December, coming in contact with so many people who have the flu, sinus infections, and chest congestion, I've been washing daily, even as a preventive after I've been out in public. At home, during the winter, along with using a humidifier, I think nose washing is keeping my nasal passages from being too dry. Usually between January and April I get a really bad sinus infection, but so far this season, not even a cold.* **❞**

Sally D., Springfield, Missouri

Heading Off Colds

❝ *Nasal washing works well for me. I use it regularly and then when I feel a cold coming on I increase the number of times each week that I use it.* **❞**

Tom R, Denver, Colorado

Finally Some Action

66 *I currently have a cold brought on by allergies. I have been washing my nose and am really starting to see the benefits. I had visited with you earlier about my ear issue, and something is moving in there - after four years! I am confident that as I continue the process, I will see more results - for now it is just having my hearing return and a cessation of the ringing. I am still amazed that the solution to my problem may be so simple.* 99

Eric P., San Diego, California

My Life is Changed. Completely.

66 *I just had to write to thank you for developing Nasopure. I've been using it now for about two years, and it has completely changed my life. I used to have nasal congestion and sinus headaches from April through late August due to seasonal allergies, and required regular use of over the counter decongestants and antihistamines just to function. This past summer I took just two antihistamines (when I was mowing several acres of lawn) and maybe five or six doses of decongestant. I also am one of those people for whom colds seem to linger on for weeks to months. Since I've been using Nasopure, though, I generally have only one bad day from a cold, and then three or four days of minor congestion, after which I'm back to normal. This product really can't be beaten for its effectiveness and ease of use. Thank you Dr. Hana for this wonderful device!* 99

Art S., St. Louis, Missouri

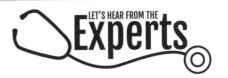

LET'S HEAR FROM THE
Experts

Warding off Colds

A cure for the common cold has been elusive. Vaccines do not work for colds because the viruses responsible for colds mutate frequently. Cold viruses and our immune systems constantly play hide-and-go-seek - viruses hiding by mutating, and our immune systems seeking their newer versions. The immune system can easily destroy cold viruses they were exposed to previously, but can we help our immune systems prevent the new ones?

Sufficient numbers of viruses are necessary to make us sick. Viruses have to enter the cell membrane lining the nose in order to replicate. They have to use our cell machinery to make new copies of viruses. They bud off these cells to spread to more cells as a cold develops. Washing the nose reduces the numbers of viruses to prevent their spread. Replication is kept at bay by washing away the new copies before they can invade more cells. Viral entry rate is the first step in determining how quickly they can make us sick. How quickly they enter is not well documented. Apparently, it is sufficiently slow to make nasal washing effective. Routine washing of the nose each day prevents viral build up. This keeps colds so minor as to be virtually undetectable by nasal washer advocates. Those washing their nose once or twice daily report rarely getting sick with colds any more. Those who feel a cold coming on can wash their nose more frequently and find symptoms disappear quickly.

Hand washing can reduce the transmission of cold viruses from hand to nose. These viruses spread by sneezing and nasal washing dramatically reduces sneezing. Well-mannered people cover their mouth and nose when they sneeze. Even if they do this with a handkerchief instead of their hand, this act still transfers viruses from noses or tissues to hands. Washing hands decreases this transfer to surfaces that are frequently touched, like doorknobs, phones, computer keyboards, shopping carts and other hands. However, people touch itchy noses more frequently than any objects. Thus, without a clean un-itchy nose, even washed hands remain infection spreaders. Those who care for children who are coughing and sneezing are particularly susceptible to viral transfers. The only sensible solution is for everyone to wash their nose routinely to flush out these virulent invaders. By this means, viral transfers by air and hand, are minimized.

When Your Defense Is Down

The Center for Disease Control (CDC) currently recommends hand washing and avoiding sick people. This is good advice. However, parents of sick children and health care professionals cannot avoid sick people. In our hectic world, people cannot skip work for a cold and children cannot skip school for colds without creating gaps in their education. For those who are ill for other reasons, a cold can be the straw that breaks the camel's back and keeps them home. For most of us, we keep right on trucking. Personally, I find washing my nose daily means I rarely catch colds and for that I am very grateful.

Marilyn James-Kracke, PhD
Associate Professor Medical Pharmacology and Physiology
University of Missouri-Columbia

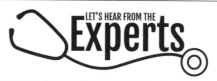

A Pharmacist's View of Nasal Washing to Treat Congestion

I work in a retail pharmacy setting serving a broad cross-section of my community's population: city dwellers, rural farming folk, young and elderly, laborers, office workers and people from several other countries around the world. As a pharmacist I have many customers approaching me about allergy problems, sinus headaches, repeated sinus infections, colds and coughs, etc.; some with acute problems, others with long-standing or recurring conditions.

My approach is to listen to their concerns and then to explain the pros and cons of a variety of approaches to help them deal with their particular problem. I will always include a more natural approach (for example, nose washing) for their consideration along with information on various allergy or other medications that might be appropriate for resolving their particular respiratory health problem.

Some customers just want the regular "cold remedy" or "sinus / congestion medication" and don't want to think about or consider a different approach. Others don't think they could deal with the "yuck" factor of nasal irrigation, especially when they're already feeling bad. But I hope that in at least mentioning the positive aspects of nasal irrigation they will perhaps consider it again at a later stage.

Then there are those customers who have tried "everything" and wonder whether there is anything else which would help, or perhaps something more natural. Pregnant women who very rightly don't want to take any medication which would hurt their growing baby are often delighted to hear about how nasal irrigation can help them better cope with their nasal symptoms. Very often it is the young husband looking for relief for his wife who comes into the pharmacy to inquire about what could be done to help.

Mothers with younger children are often happily surprised that nasal irrigation is something that they can safely use to decrease their child's allergy symptoms, or cough and cold - naturally with little to no adverse effects. This information is especially useful for these young parents since the latest warnings from the Food and Drug Administration to avoid using over-the-counter cold and flu remedies on children under six years of age.

Once people understand the logic and simplicity of nasal irrigation they are usually keen to at least try the technique. I have feedback from customers who use nasal irrigation regularly and swear by it, saying that it has decreased their allergy symptoms, has shortened the length and severity of a cold and seems to have helped in preventing the development of some secondary upper respiratory infections and decreasing their sinus infections.

I too have used nose washing to help me with sinus or nasal problems and can vouch for the benefits of using this simple medical approach. It is very easy to prepare the nose washing solution and very easy to do the actual nose washing. The procedure is very easy on the body and works very well with respiratory medications for allergies and congestion.

Muriel Vincent, Pharmacist
Columbia, Missouri

A Believer

Sinus Problems and Bacterial Infections

Chronic Sinusitis

✓ Chronic sinusitis is one of the most commonly diagnosed chronic illnesses in the United States, affecting forty to fifty million Americans each year.

✓ Chronic sinusitis begins with an inflammation of the mucous membranes in your sinuses. This inflammation causes fluid buildup, eventually plugging the sinus cavity and preventing normal mucus drainage.

✓ Chronic sinusitis can be a miserable condition that significantly impairs your quality of life. If you have chronic sinusitis, you may have difficulty breathing through your nose or experience frequent headaches and tenderness in the face or aching behind the eyes. You may also have frequent yellow or greenish discharge from your nose or drainage down the back of your throat.

✓ Chronic sinusitis can be caused by infections of the upper respiratory tract - the nose, pharynx, sinuses and throat - but there are noninfectious triggers also. Allergies are a common cause, and anatomical problems such as a deviated nasal septum or polyps can bring on chronic sinusitis.

✓ Although most cases of sinusitis clear up in less than four weeks (termed "acute"), when the condition recurs or lasts longer than twelve consecutive weeks, you have developed a case of chronic sinusitis.

✓ Chronic sinusitis may be caused by mold or fungi in the sinuses.

✓ Research suggests that nasal irrigation is useful in the treatment of chronic sinusitis, with improvements in sinus-related quality of life, decreases in symptoms and decreases medication use.

✓ Symptoms include bad breath, fatigue, lack of concentration, difficulty kissing, and depression.

Biofilm is a covering, a film, often stuck to the membranes much like plaque on the teeth or the slippery slime on river stones. This bacterial community consists of two major components: bacteria and the body's white cells (the cells which fight infections). Biofilm is often stuck to the mucosal linings and is very difficult to remove. More than 99% of all bacteria live in biofilm communities. Some are beneficial, but biofilm can cause problems. Antibiotics kill or inhibit bacteria but if the bacteria are within a biofilm, the antibiotic may not necessarily reach them. Often, these films can be physically removed by simply washing them away. See page 80 on Biofilms!

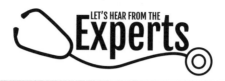
Known causes of headaches are pressure points in the nose made more intense by nasal swelling. We have relieved many severe chronic headaches simply by encouraging our patients to use buffered hypertonic nasal saline irrigation regularly. The solution pulls the excess water from the swollen membranes, thereby relieving the nasal swelling that intensifies the pressure point. This often cures the headache.

David S. Parsons, MD,
FAAP, FACSClinical Professor,
Universities of North and South Carolina
Pediatric Otolaryngology, Charlotte Eye, Ear,
Nose and Throat Associates

Chronic Sinusitis Gone

❝ *When I first came in touch with Dr. Hana's Nasopure system, I had such significant nasal and allergy issues that I had almost given up hope of a life free of daily medications and yearly antibiotics from chronic sinus infections. Within a matter of months of using the rinse twice daily, I was able to both give up my daily antihistamine and decongestant routine, as well as happily discontinue my presence at the doctor's office for sinus infections. It is hard for me to find the adequate words to describe my gratitude, appreciation and admiration for Dr. Hana and her no-nonsense, straightforward approach to relieving chronic nasal issues which had plagued me almost daily for over twenty-five years.* **❞**

Grady Pope, Cambria, California

After Years, Easy Breathing

66 *I've suffered with chronic sinusitis for years and have tried many, many treatments with mixed results, none lasting. I have already noticed my breathing through my nose seems much easier since I began my nasal rinsing!* **99**

Michael L. Collins, RN, Leavenworth, Kansas

Sinus Infection-Free

66 *I do recommend nasal washing to anyone who complains of sinus infections. I seldom suffer from one anymore. I am 100% sold on regular nasal washing. Since I started three years ago, I have not had one sinus infection. Before then I was getting one to three sinus infections a year for at least ten years.* **99**

Jo C., Charleston, West Virginia

I Trusted My Doctor

66 *My physician recommended nasal washing for my allergies and sinus headaches. I was reluctant at first but eventually decided to give it a try. My experience has been nothing but positive. I breathe much better and do not need to use nasal sprays half as much. Thank you!* **99**

Rosanne B, Springfield, Massachusetts

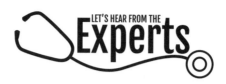

Sinusitis and Nasal Lavage (Washing)

I have practiced internal medicine for many years in academic settings. Early in my career I became aware of nasal lavage (washing) solutions for patients with allergies and recurrent sinus infections. However, in those days, ways to deliver a good lavage were limited and there was little in the medical literature to verify the benefits. So I prescribed this for a few patients but did not promote it for wide-scale use. About six years ago, three changes occurred that have influenced my thinking about nasal lavage.

First of all, I personally started getting recurrent sinus infections and a worsening of my allergies (which probably contributed to the infections). Secondly, after moving to Columbia, Missouri, working at the University of Missouri Health Care, I heard about the Nasopure nasal lavage system. I contacted Dr. Solomon for more information and was able to meet with her to learn more. I was impressed with her commitment to promote nasal lavage.

I decided to start using it myself. It was easy to use but I must admit that I would try it for few days and then forget about it. However, after getting over yet another sinus infection, I was determined to use it on a regular basis and have done so (using it at least once per day) ever since. One cannot draw general scientific conclusions from one person's experience but I have found that the frequency of my infections has decreased dramatically.

Third, medical studies started to come out showing the benefits of nasal lavage. This has been gratifying because it is normally very difficult to find funding for this type of research and I laud the efforts of the investigators in this area.

To me it is clear that nasal lavage is very useful for patients with allergies or sinusitis. Lavage can lessen the need for medications. The problem is getting the patient to use lavage regularly, as my personal experience has shown.

I have found the following tips helpful:

1. *Carefully educate the patient on the benefits of nasal lavage. I frequently compare it with the importance of hand washing.*

2. *Address any concerns such as the often expressed fear that it will go into their ears.*

3. *If you use it yourself as I do, let them know that.*

4. *Tell them to keep the bottle in the shower or on the edge of the tub so that they can't miss it before bathing. This also has the advantage of allowing the solution to drain while in the shower.*

5. *On return visits, ask them how their use of saline lavage is working for them. Keep encouraging its use.*

6. *Recommend that nasal lavage be performed daily, even (or especially) on vacation. Using on long plane rides can also be very beneficial.*

In summary, I feel that every patient with allergies or recurrent sinus infections should be given the opportunity to try saline lavage. With encouragement from their care providers, they will hopefully find it of benefit and will continue to use it regularly.

Robert Hodge, MD, FACP, FACPE, CPE
Past Chair of Internal Medicine
University Medical Center, University of Missouri, Columbia, Missouri

Free of Infection

66 *I noticed after using nose rinses faithfully all one spring, I didn't have even one sinus infection. The previous spring I had been treated with three antibiotics! It really seems to help with upper respiratory infection control.* 99

Kathy I., Registered Nurse, Albuquerque, New Mexico

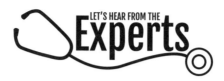

A Naturopathic Approach to Sinus Issues

When treating sinus-related conditions with a naturopathic approach, symptomatic relief is an important goal, but even more important is treatment of the actual cause. When the deeper cause is treated, symptoms subsequently clear up and the resulting relief is more effective and lasting.

Hydrotherapy, the use of different temperatures of water in a variety of applications, provides many potential benefits. These techniques can help equally in the healing of both infectious and allergic related conditions.

One simple hydrotherapy technique is nasal irrigation. Originating in many cultures historically, it is best known from the Ayurvedic tradition of ancient India. The simple process of washing out the nose can have great results both in the treatment of many common sinus related conditions as well as a preventive measure.

This technique is based on basic principles of hygiene. To perform this procedure, one mixes salt into warm purified water to make a saline solution. This solution is then used to wash out the sinuses. A traditional "neti" pot can be used, or there are a number of user friendly devices available on the market. These modernized versions often employ a squeeze bottle or syringe type device that many of my patients find easier and more convenient than the traditional "neti" pot. Any of these devices can be helpful; the most important thing is consistent use.

Another easy and effective hydrotherapy technique gives profound relief to the congestive pain and pressure of inflamed sinus passages. Application of alternating hot and cold moist compresses can offer relief to throbbing and inflamed sinus passages. It acts to pump interstitial fluids away from the area, reducing inflammation while bringing increased blood flow and increased white blood cell activity.

> *By combining a variety of natural approaches to relieve symptoms and assist the body's healing process while treating the underlying dysfunctions, the naturopathic approach can bring about powerful and lasting relief to many common sinus-related conditions.*
>
> Mark Green, Naturopathic Doctor
> Overland Park, Kansas

Natural Remedy

❝ *I had begun suffering from chronic sinus infections on a regular basis and was constantly on medication in attempt to alleviate the symptoms. Not liking the idea of being medicated on a continual basis, I was open to any options available to me, except surgery. Shortly after nasal washing was introduced, my daughter mentioned it to me and I was very open to the idea of using natural ingredients to cure the infections. I immediately began feeling better and my infections disappeared. I now wash my nose daily and also immediately after doing any yard work.* **❞**

Viole Columbia, Missouri

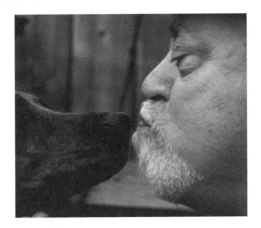

Finally Free of Drug-Resistant Infections

❝ *I am a 30-year-old man who spent four years dealing with chronic sinus infections. I don't like to take antibiotics, but I did - over and over again. My infection was caused by MRSA and it took expensive medications to treat it. So that's what I did - took the medicine which made me feel a little better, but every time I finished the antibiotics, they would culture my sinuses and the culture stayed positive for MRSA. I was unwilling to stay on antibiotics all the time. Finally, the last time I was really sick, instead of using antibiotics I washed with hypertonic saline four times a day for a solid three weeks. And finally, for the first time in four years, my culture was negative at the end of that three weeks. And I have been free of infection ever since. You have no idea how happy I am! Thank you thank you thank you!* **❞**

David S, Los Angeles, California

Fungal Sinusitis

 Fungi are infectious living organisms that are different from viral or bacterial particles. Is there a fungus among us? Yes there is! Our normal human bodies contain many fungi as part of the natural balance of microbes (flora) in the intestines. The interesting point to remember about fungi is that they live and coexist in a natural balance with other microorganisms that colonize our bodies. But under certain conditions, fungi overpower the balance, causing a mild infection or even a life-threatening episode.

Fungal infections are more likely to increase with the use of antibiotics. This is because antibiotics encourage the overproduction of fungi by killing not only bad bacteria, but also the good bacteria that keep our microflora in balance.

Thousands of kinds of single-cell fungi (molds and yeasts) are found everywhere in the world. Fungal spores (the reproductive part of the organism) become airborne like pollen and some people develop allergies to fungi. When fungi cause inflammation or infection of the sinuses, it is termed *fungal sinusitis*. Despite the tens of thousands of fungal types, human illnesses are related to only a few dozen varieties.

Though infections of the nose and sinus *(rhino sinusitis)* are a common disorder, the role of fungus in chronic sinusitis remains unclear. There seem to be more questions than answers.

By far the most common type of fungus infection in the sinuses is "allergic fungal sinusitis" but the rarest and most serious is the chronic invasive sinusitis. Although this is not a true allergic reaction, it is a reaction of the immune system. Occasionally, inflammation leads to destruction of bony tissue, causing blockage of normal mucus drainage and resulting in a difficult road toward successful treatment. Re-establishment of normal sinus drainage with removal of the fungi is the first step in treatment.

Due to the long term inflammation which is often present, nasal polyps are frequently associated with this condition. These polyps then contribute to a vicious cycle of inability to keep the mucus flowing. Extended or lifelong medical and intermittent surgical management is often required. Treatment routes are still controversial but they do include surgery, steroids, antihistamines, antibiotics, anti-fungal medications, allergy immunotherapy and of course, regular irrigations.

It is clear that millions in the United States suffer from chronic sinusitis and up until a few years ago, fungal sources were thought to be the culprit in the majority of cases. However, there is a rising tide from the experts that not all chronic infections are fungal. Rather, many are related to dysfunction of cilia, overuse of antibiotics, past medication use, chronic allergies, and diabetes.

Drainage, cleaning, and irrigation are the first steps in treatment of any chronic sinusitis. In fact, if this is not done, all the drugs in the world cannot help.

Toxic Mold

> 66 *I work in a clinic in Kansas City and received a nose wash as a gift. It was wonderful. I've been using it ever since. I was told by my doctor that I have a large perforated septum as result of Toxic Mold Syndrome. Irrigating my nasal passages has been the only thing that has caused the daily bleeding, discomfort and crustiness to cease. Thank you.* 99

Traci B, Kansas City, Missouri

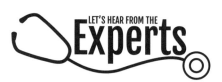
LET'S HEAR FROM THE Experts

Antibiotics have long been used to treat the bacteria that cause sinus infections. Studies show that antibiotics benefit both acute and chronic sinusitis. However, the benefit in either case is surprisingly minimal and lasts only about a week at best. There are hazards of antibiotics as well. First, antibiotics promote overgrowth of antibiotic-resistant bacteria, requiring the use of more potent (and expensive) antibiotics the next time. At the same time, antibiotics also greatly suppress healthy bacteria. Each person has on the order of a billion "good" bacteria that normally populate the nose and throat. These normal bacteria almost surely keep infectious bacteria in check. It may take roughly six weeks to re-populate the area after it has been depleted by a course of antibiotics. So, at least theoretically, one approach is to simply stop using antibiotics for a period of at least six weeks. This can usually be done provided the person does not encounter any unusually severe episodes. The value of this approach has never been studied, but it certainly seems sensible.

Michael Cooperstock, MD, MPH
Pediatric Infectious Disease
University of Missouri, Columbia, Medical Center

Allergies and Hay Fever

Allergic Rhinitis (head congestion, sneezing, tearing, and swelling of the nasal mucous membranes caused by an allergic reaction) is what most people refer to as *hay fever*. This is the fifth most common chronic illness in the United States, affecting tens of millions of Americans, resulting in dramatic costs in lost productivity and dollars spent. Hay fever causes millions of people to miss work or school each year. The total cost is in the billions each year. Doctors write some forty million prescriptions every year for allergic rhinitis; in addition, most people who do purchase non-prescription medications buy them in an attempt to relieve their symptoms.

In 2003, the journal *Pediatric Allergy and Immunology* published a study that supported the use of nasal irrigation with hypertonic saline as a preventative option in seasonal allergic rhinitis-related symptoms in the pediatric patient. Twenty children with seasonal allergic rhinitis to a specific weed were enrolled in the study. Ten children were randomized to receive three times daily nasal irrigation with hypertonic saline for the entire pollen season, which lasted six weeks. Ten patients were to receive no nasal irrigation and were used as the controls. A daily log based on the presence of nasal itching, nasal discharge (rhinorrhea), nasal obstruction and sneezing was tabulated for each week of the pollen season. These children used antihistamines as needed and recorded each dose. In patients using nasal irrigation, after two weeks of nasal washing the daily nasal complaints decreased and after three weeks this reduction was statistically significant. With the decrease in symptoms, fewer antihistamines were consumed. These effects became more evident with continued use of nasal washes.

This particular study supports the use of nasal irrigation with hypertonic saline in the pediatric patient with seasonal allergic rhinitis. The researchers reported that this approach was tolerable, inexpensive and effective.

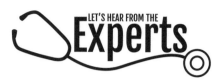
LET'S HEAR FROM THE
Experts

Allergies and the Nose

When talking about allergies, regardless of the situation, it is repeated exposure that causes sensitivity. It doesn't matter if you are talking about bee stings or Brussels sprouts - if an allergic-prone individual is exposed to an antigen enough times, they are going to reach their threshold and manifest symptoms - whatever those symptoms may be.

An example that I often use in talking with patients is that of a glass half full of liquid - in a non-allergic individual, you can pour in anything- pollen, dust mites, peanuts, etc. - and the cup will remain half full. In an allergic individual, however, when allergens start pouring in, the liquid level rises and at some point will overflow and the patient will show symptoms. Thus, much of the advice I give patients centers on how to keep their particular cup from overflowing, by controlling the things that they realistically can.

We can't control what the pollen count is going to be outside but we certainly can exercise control over our home's interior environment by keeping the windows shut and cleaning the home thoroughly and regularly. After being outside we can wash our noses, thus dislodging the pollen and mold that may have landed on the nasal mucosa, and preventing the allergic cascade from starting. We can use good judgment in what we eat - limiting processed foods with artificial flavors, colors, chemicals, etc. and filling ourselves with as much real food as possible. Regular exercise and stress reduction also play important roles in the immune system's function and good health.

When most people contemplate their nose, they generally don't think of it as being the part of their lungs/respiratory system that they can see. The nose is, in fact, the beginning of the respiratory system, and its health is crucial to having a healthy operating respiratory system. That is why it is especially important for asthmatics to keep their noses in good operating condition, because if the nose is inflamed, it will translate into lung tissue being inflamed.

> *The nose is the first line of defense for the lungs against the outside world - whether it is pollen, chemicals, or viruses - and the healthier the nose is kept, the better the lungs will function.*

Laurie Fowler, MD
Allergy and Immunology, Pediatrics
Columbia, Missouri

A Healthy Step

❝ *Spring allergy symptoms were much better with a daily wash earlier this year, and I just recovered from my first cold in over two years. Twice daily irrigation was a huge help in relieving congestion. (To be blunt, I couldn't believe the quantity of gunk that came out with irrigation, and that was after the traditional 'dry' blow stopped yielding.)*

Here's another way to say it: in almost a year of use, I have not gone to bed once with a clogged nose. The positive impact on sleep quality is hard to overstate. Besides taking up running, nasal washing is the best personal health step I've taken this year. **❞**

James B, Sartell, Minnesota

Experts

Saline Irrigation and Allergic Rhinitis

Allergic rhinitis is a prevalent, expensive and often frustrating condition with major impact on the quality of life and daily functioning of those who suffer. A significant proportion of allergic rhinitis patients develop complications such as asthma, chronic or recurrent sinusitis and nasal polyposis (multiple polyps). While the underlying bodily changes of acute allergic inflammation mediated by certain antibodies is well understood, physicians are not sure how the treatments really change the outcome. There is increasing evidence that nasal saline irrigation may play a beneficial role in additional or supportive management of allergies of the nose and sinuses.

Allergic patients may suffer seasonally, perennially, or both, depending on their sensitization patterns. There are three distinct pollen seasons in North America - tree, grass, and weed. Year-round airborne allergens (particles which cause troublesome reactions) include dust mites, pet dander and certain mold spores. A person cannot develop an allergic response to a particular irritant without being exposed at least once, and then exposed again to that same irritant. This explains why infants cannot be allergic to pollen in their first year or season of life. An allergic response occurs when specific antibodies trigger a sequence of chemical reactions which affect blood vessels, nerves and glands to produce the classic symptoms of sneezing, itchy watery eyes and nose, and congestion.

The highest percentage of people with allergies are kids; 40%, compared with 20% of adults. Treating allergies is expensive. The most recent estimates of the overall costs for allergic rhinitis exceed ten billion dollars per year, making it one of the most expensive chronic illnesses of American patients. However, those figures could be much lower than the actual costs. Despite the discomfort of the disease, fewer than 15% of allergy sufferers seek specific treatment from healthcare providers, often preferring non-prescription and self-administered therapies.

The conventional management of allergies includes educating patients about controlling their environment, drug therapy to prevent and/or relieve symptoms and allergy shots for severe cases. However, these standard approaches are not as effective as doctors or patients would like. Avoiding exposure to allergens (controlling one's environment) is quite difficult for patients who experience allergy-related symptoms several months of the year. In addition, almost all medications merely treat symptoms and do not provide long-term reduction of the underlying disease. And although allergy shots may slow the progression of symptoms, a regimen of shots requires a significant time commitment, is initially expensive and demands close observation for possible reactions. Obviously, it is important to find better ways to treat the many people who suffer from nasal/sinus allergies.

The benefit of saline nasal irrigation as an additional therapy for various sinus disorders is well-described in the medical literature. The procedure flushes the nasal cavity, which promotes the evacuation of allergen and irritant-containing mucus secretions. A recent Cochrane collaborative report identified eight trials in patients with chronic rhino sinusitis, comparing nasal irrigation and other active therapies or placebo. The authors concluded that this procedure is valuable as supportive therapy in many sinus patients, regardless of the underlying cause of the inflammation.

There are several randomized, controlled trials of saline irrigation in seasonal or perennial allergic rhinitis. One of the largest is a study of 40 grass-allergic Italian children, half of whom received nasal rinsing three times a day during a seven week pollen season. Compared to children not using irrigation, the treated patients had lower symptom scores and markedly reduced intake of oral antihistamines. Thus, saline irrigation appears effective, safe and well-tolerated even in children with long term symptoms from allergic rhinitis.

Specific mechanisms underlying beneficial effects of nasal lavage are not completely understood. Several factors affect the underlying disease process, which explains why nasal washing works. First, there is obviously a direct cleansing effect of the saline as it flushes out irritants and removes obstructive mucoid secretions. Second, studies have shown that washing actually removes the cells which cause nasal and sinus problems. Third, washing with saline solution improves the cilia-beating mechanism in the nasal system.

In conclusion, allergic rhinitis is a common debilitating and often under-treated disorder with major impact on health costs and quality of life. There are significant drawbacks associated with all existing therapies, leaving room for complementary approaches. Nasal saline irrigation has been shown to be effective in reducing symptoms and medication usage; is safe and well tolerated even in young children, and is relatively inexpensive, especially compared to prescription treatment. This technique should be considered for many allergic rhinitis patients and further study is warranted to determine if nasal irrigation can prevent chronic illness from sinusitis, nasal polyps and possibly asthma.

Mark Vandewalker, MD
Asthma and Allergy Consultants
Columbia, Missouri

Avoiding the Prescriptions

66 *I am an allergy sufferer in California. I love where I live, but I do suffer from allergies to everything in this county except redwoods and eucalyptus. I wash my nose after I work in my yard or when the wind blows grass and pollen around so much that I can't avoid it. This past weekend I went to a party that was so much fun I forgot my allergies. The party was held in a converted greenhouse in the middle of a field and it was a windy day. We played games and in one of the games I was*

*challenged to put two marigolds up my nose and cry out, 'USA!
USA!' In the spirit of the moment, I performed this act and
everyone laughed. I never thought about marigolds up my nose
along with dust, grass, pollen, chicken manure particles and
goat hairs.*

*I remembered my allergies the next day when I had such sinus
congestion that I could hardly breathe out of my right nostril. I
felt horrible. I started rinsing with saline solution immediately
and did it several times that day. I was pretty certain that I
would have a sinus infection because that is what always
happens when I get this congested, but I was willing to try
rinsing aggressively first because I hate taking medications.*

*This morning I could breathe, and although I am still getting
dark discharge out with the help of nasal rinsing, I think I am
going to avoid antibiotics after all!* **"**

Cynthia W., Willits, California

Wash Those Allergies Out

" *Here in Sonoma County, California wine country we have
a significant problem with allergies. It rarely freezes in our area
so allergies can often be a year-round problem. If it's not pollen,
it's the vineyards, or the dust, or the mold we get from living so
close to the foggy Pacific coast.*

*Many of my family practice patients are true allergy sufferers
but would like to avoid using daily medication to manage their
symptoms. Prevention is always preferable to treatment! I too
am an allergy sufferer, and several years ago was taught nasal
rinsing by my own ENT specialist after having surgery on my*

sinuses. Since that time I have been teaching the nasal wash technique and encouraging my patients to adopt this as part of their daily hygiene.

Once patients feel the benefits of a clear nose, they are only too willing to continue treating their sinus and allergy symptoms using this very natural method. **99**

Stacey M. Kerr, MD, Santa Rosa, California

Sore Throats: "My Throat Is Killing Me"

We have all experienced that troublesome tickle in the throat, a burning or scratching sensation, or the sore throat associated with infections of strep or mono *(mononucleosis)*. Sore throats can be due to many things. Causes include viruses (common cold, mononucleosis), bacteria *(Streptococcus pharyngitis)*, smoking, breathing polluted air, drinking alcohol, allergies and sinus drainage, just to mention a few.

The most common cause of a mild tickle or scratchy throat is due to annoying mucus. Allergies and viruses both cause increased production of mucus. Mucus is acidic, so you can imagine that when this substance drains down the back of the throat and is allowed to sit there, it can be painful. Most often the pain is worse in the morning and gets a little better as the day progresses. Why? The drainage drips down the throat during sleep and one awakens with a really sore throat. As we eat, drink and swallow the mucus begins to clear away from the tender membranes that line the throat, allowing the inflamed tissues to quiet down again.

Sometimes breathing through the mouth will cause a sore throat in the absence of any infection. During the months of dry winter air, some people will often wake up with a sore throat. This usually disappears after having something to drink.

In addition, stomach reflux can result in a painful throat. If the acidic contents of the stomach reflux up high enough to irritate the throat, it can cause a persistent cough and sore throat. This is more common than you might think.

Tonsillitis refers to swelling, inflammation, and infection of the tonsils. These collections or "balls of lymph tissue" live behind your tongue, one on either side of your throat. These solid tissue masses have crevices (like a dried prune) which can harbor infections as well as food debris. Tonsils often peak in size during late childhood at seven to ten years of age, and usually shrink in size after this time. Allergies or chronic sinus infections may contribute to the persistence of enlarged tonsils. This makes sense since tonsils are reactive tissues; they filter and they respond to irritants, and they enlarge when exposed to infections. The size alone does not necessarily cause pain but the presence of white cells and other components that respond to infections *(exudates)* will. Additionally, large tonsils can affect voice quality, taste and smell. One can also experience what feels like a swelling or sense of fullness in the throat. Signs of strep throat (bacterial infection) and tonsillitis (general term for infection of the tonsils) are often alike. Bacteria usually cause tonsillitis, though sometimes a virus or even an abscess (local infection of one single tonsil) may be involved.

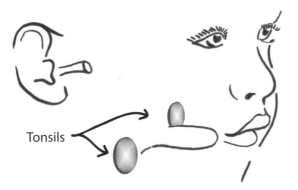

Tonsils

Signs and Symptoms of Tonsillitis or Strep Throat:

✓ Sore throat, pain when swallowing.

✓ Fever and chills.

✓ Fatigue.

✓ Headaches.

✓ Vomiting (mainly in kids).

✓ White patches on tonsils, beefy red tonsils or tiny red dots on the soft palate.

✓ Sore glands in neck and jaw.

✓ Ear pain.

✓ Decreased appetite.

✓ Creases in the skin (elbows, stomach folds) turn red (*pastia lines*).

✓ Faint rash on trunk (*Scarlet Fever*).

✓ Strep throat is usually *not* associated with preceding sinus congestion, cold or allergy symptoms. Strep will "hit you like a ton of bricks;" one minute you are fine, the next you are feeling very ill.

The only reason to remove the tonsils is severe and/or recurrent tonsillitis, or if the airway becomes obstructed.

The Scoop on Strep

One caveat from my clinical experience is this: Parents often bring their children in for a strep test and treatment within what seems like hours of their child's first complaint. The tests are not 100% accurate during the early stages of this illness but if tested on day two or three, these tests are much more reliable.

Often, doctors will treat the patient with antibiotics despite a negative strep test, thinking the test may be giving a false negative and wanting to be on the safe side. This is an issue if we are trying to prevent antibiotic overuse, resistance, or side effects. In addition, I have found that if a viral sore throat is inappropriately treated with antibiotics, more often than not a rash develops. Then we wonder: is that rash from a virus, from a virus interacting with an antibiotic or because of an allergic reaction to the drug? The resulting unnecessary confusion can affect a child's health history and treatments for years to come.

Today, people seem to develop strep on a recurring basis. Forty years ago, if one was ill, the patient was not treated until many days into the illness. I suspect that this, although not pleasant for the patient or family, actually allowed the body to develop antibodies against the strep bacteria, so if exposed months or years later, the patient did not develop the illness. That explains, perhaps, why adults develop strep less frequently as compared to children. Conversely, if strep is treated within twenty-four hours, the body's antibodies do not have an opportunity to develop.

When you're certain it's strep, use the antibiotics! Strep is treated to prevent the spread of infection that could damage heart valves or cause other complications. But throat infections caused by most viruses (which can be extremely painful as well) are treated symptomatically: rest, fluids, warm soups and drinks, frequent gargles with warm salt water. Popsicles, hard candies or throat lozenges can be very soothing, because they increase saliva production, but should not be used in very young children because of the risk of choking.

Of course, no matter what the cause of the sore throat, medications can treat symptoms but washing the nasal passages will reduce the bulk of the mucus drainage, if present.

A Believer

66 *I first heard of nasal washing from a physician who said 'the simple prophylactic habit of nose douching should be routine.' I returned home from a trip to Japan about twelve days ago; three days later I came down with a severe sore throat. It was not strep. The doctor recommended Mucinex and continued practice of nasal washing. She did predict that even with this* *regimen the sore throat would last six-seven days. Sure enough, the sore throat vanished on the sixth day and the virus has been defeated. So, I am a believer. Nasal washing works.* **99**

JoAnn M., Reno, Nevada

Post-Nasal Drip

Post-nasal drip is mucus accumulation in the back of the nose and throat resulting in mucus dripping downward from the back of the nose. One of the most common characteristics of inflammation of the inner lining of the nose *(chronic rhinitis)* is post-nasal drip. Sometimes, in my office, we call this "Toxic Snot Syndrome." Post-nasal drip can be caused by excessive or thick secretions or impairment in the normal clearance of mucus from the nose and throat. This annoying drip may lead to chronic sore throats, a persistent cough, or that familiar and frequent habit of clearing your throat.

Daily nose washing can relieve and, in time, eliminate the symptoms and causes of post-nasal drip.

What a Relief

66 *For many years, upon waking up in the morning, I would cough for at least 30 minutes due to what my physician diagnosed as post-nasal drip. I learned about nasal washing eight months ago and thought that I would give it a try. By washing my nose each evening and morning, I no longer cough! It makes my life so much better.* **99**

Ethel O., Pensacola, Florida

I Didn't Even Know There Was Anything Wrong

❝ *What I want to share is what is happening just in one day of washing. I have never known my nose was not clear, it always seemed clear, but I now know that is was far from clear. I am breathing easier, I feel things moving around in my ear canal, and the most impressive part is that I awoke this morning to find no mucus in my throat or ears, and when I got up and rinsed my mouth, there was no weird brown stuff that usually comes out of my mouth. And my throat feels better than it has in years. I could still taste my toothpaste, which never happens, ever, always a nasty foul smelling brown, yuck. I think I have had these issues for so long, I was not even aware of it, or that it could be different.* ❞

Paul S, Cincinnati, Ohio

So Very Grateful for the Simple Solution

❝ *I must tell you that I have been dealing with mucus in my throat for months, and nothing was getting it under control. I put one ounce of the hypertonic solution through each nostril this morning and that mucus and irritation is gone. I have no words. Such a simple thing, and I am aware of its importance, but did not realize the full gravity of it. Thank you, the world needs this. I cannot wait until next week to begin introducing them to my clients.* ❞

Gary Y, Nutritionist, Portland Oregon

Constant Runny Nose (Vasomotor Rhinitis)

Vasomotor rhinitis is also known as non-allergenic rhinitis, because it often has the same nasal symptoms as allergies, but has different causes. While allergic rhinitis conditions, such as hay fever and dust allergies are the result of the immune system overreacting to environmental irritants (pollen, etc), vasomotor rhinitis is believed to be caused by oversensitive or excessive blood vessels in the nasal membranes. These blood vessels, which are controlled in turn by the autonomic nervous system, either constrict or dilate in order to regulate mucus flow and congestion. Vasomotor rhinitis is a common condition that often goes unrecognized or under-recognized. An estimated seventeen million Americans have vasomotor rhinitis.

People who suffer from vasomotor rhinitis experience an overreaction to stimuli such as changes in weather, temperature or barometric pressure. These individuals react to chemical irritants like smoke, ozone, pollution, perfumes and aerosol sprays, psychological stress and emotional shocks, certain types of medications, alcohol, and even spicy food. So while a normal person's nose may run on a very cold day, a vasomotor rhinitis sufferer's nose may start running (or go completely dry) simply by walking into a slightly colder (or slightly warmer) room, or from eating food that is slightly warmer or cooler than room temperature. While a normal person may tolerate a certain degree of cigarette smoke, the vasomotor rhinitis sufferer may experience significant discomfort from the same level of smoke.

Vasomotor rhinitis appears to be significantly more common in women than men, leading some researchers to believe that hormones to play a role. In general, onset occurs after twenty years of age, in contrast to allergic rhinitis, which generally appears before adulthood. People suffering from vasomotor rhinitis typically experience symptoms year-round, though symptoms may be worse in the spring and fall when rapid weather changes are more common.

In my experience, the best and therefore the first treatment to relieve vasomotor rhinitis is nasal rinsing with a buffered hypertonic solution. Rinsing helps eliminate the original irritant without the side effects of medications. Washing does no harm and is tolerated well when the patient is taught the proper technique.

Cough, Cough, Cough

 In addition to a sore throat, post-nasal drip and GERD (*gastroesophageal reflux disease*, aka excessive heartburn) can cause a chronic tickling annoying cough. Here I would like to look at another kind of persistent irritating problem, the night-time cough.

This bothersome cough can really be disrupting while trying to sleep. Often a cough gets worse at night and the reason is simple. If there is sinus congestion or nasal discharge, once you lie down the secretions drip straight down the back of the throat. This drainage can result in a cough without an irritating, scratchy or painful throat.

I often receive requests for medications to treat night-time cough, but we must realize that treating is often just hiding the source, tricking the brain to stop the cough reflex. This valuable reflex actually protects our lungs. When drainage drips down the throat, the cough forces the discharge up and out into the mouth to expectorate (spit) or swallow. When the cough is suppressed with drugs, the discharge drains down into the lower airways and can infect the lungs. Using medications to suppress coughs regularly for many days or weeks can allow pneumonia to develop.

I have a guideline for my patients: use a cough suppressant for a single night but never longer without first knowing and addressing the source. Only then may cough suppressants be used but only for another two or three days (*maximum*) before bed. They should not to be used during the daytime. This ensures good sleep quality, which is vital for restoration of health, yet allows the normal and natural daytime clearance of secretions.

Common causes of nighttime cough:

- ✓ Allergies
- ✓ Sinusitis
- ✓ Post-nasal drip (from allergies, sinusitis)
- ✓ Asthma
- ✓ Croup (swelling caused by viral involvement of the vocal cords)
- ✓ COPD (chronic obstructive pulmonary disease)
- ✓ Congestive heart failure
- ✓ GERD- (Gastro esophageal reflux disease, or acid reflux). When the valve at the junction of the stomach and esophagus does not close properly, acidic contents from the stomach can back up into the esophagus and the throat causing coughing. This can also result in ear infections and sinus infections in children, as well as adults. This acid irritates the esophagus and can cause common heartburn, acid taste and coughing. Everyone experiences this on occasion, but if recurrent, it is called GERD.

When I was a resident physician still in training, the idea that GERD in children causes coughing was not known. But my mentors (Dr. Barbero and Dr. Parsons) studied this and demonstrated the relationship between GERD and cough, ear issues and asthma. This relationship had not been identified prior to their study. Infants and children normally have some degree of GERD which resolves as they age.

Finally, some medications actually can cause a dry cough, including some blood pressure meds, so you may want to check with your doctor or pharmacist to learn if this might be a problem for you.

Nose Washing Working Like a Charm

66 *I'm happy to report that nose washing is working like a charm. I coughed much less the first few days and I rarely cough at all anymore. I do it as a part of a routine like brushing my teeth.* **99**

Barbara B., Phoenix, Arizona

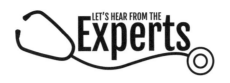

A critical therapy for reflux is the diet: no caffeine (caffeine is in coffee, tea, chocolate and colas), no mints, no acidic beverages, no tobacco or alcohol, and nothing to eat within two to three hours of lying down. We tell our patients that "decaf" means caffeine is present. Decaf means less caffeine, not no caffeine, so all coffees contain caffeine. There are three types of tea: regular, decaf (both of which have caffeine) and herbal (no caffeine). Chocolate also comes in three major types: dark and milk (lots of caffeine) and white (no caffeine). Colas are bad for two reasons: many contain caffeine but all are carbonated. Carbonation causes belching and belching is reflux. Mints relax the valve at the top of the stomach allowing reflux to occur. If this is not successful, we ask our patients to try a low carbohydrate diet for a period of several weeks and longer if there is good success. None of these therapies cost money and they are successful in patients who will follow the diet instructions!

David S. Parsons, MD, FAAP, FACS Clinical Professor, Universities of North and South Carolina Pediatric Otolaryngology, Charlotte Eye, Ear, Nose and Throat Associates

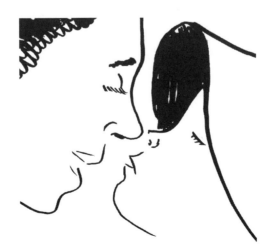

Chronic Cough Now History

> 66 *I get a chronic, annoying cough during the winter that usually lasts anywhere from four to six months. I've gone to allergists, ENTs, family physicians and nothing makes my cough go away. I've been diagnosed with non-allergic rhinosinusitis but I just think I have chronic post nasal drip. I like nasal washing because I can do it in the shower. After many years of my chronic cough, I have found that nasal washing finally got rid of it.* 99

Mike J., Portsmouth, New Hampshire

Please No More Doctor Visits!

> 66 *I have dealt with allergies for years, and can usually bring them under control before I get sick. I do not like taking medicine to treat the symptoms, and always prefer the holistic approach whenever I can learn of one.*

My first experience with Nasopure was last spring when the allergies, oak in particular, began tickling my nose. Something was in the air. Overnight I was clogged up and coughing, just plain sick. But instead of being able to control it with my other rinse, the cough quickly escalated and was now deep in my chest, cough and with fever.

So I did what I dread. I went to the doctor, was told I had bronchitis, and was prescribed a steroid and some cough medicine. That worked pretty well, but at the end of the ten days my cough was not gone. I called to get a refill on the meds. It was so upsetting to be told I would have to come back for another office visit.

At that point, my dear sweet husband went online and was lead to your site. After visiting with you, he ordered the Nasopure. It began clearing me up immediately and within one week my coughing was down to nothing and I was well on my way to recovery, without any more medicine!

It is now part of my daily regimen. I have never found anything that could kept me breathing clear and healthy like the Nasopure. When the pollens are high, and I begin to feel the effects, I rinse several times a day. Our whole family is now using the Nasopure on a daily basis. **99**

Dian W, Nashville, Tennessee

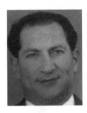

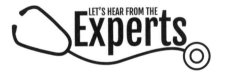

LET'S HEAR FROM THE

Covering Your Mouth Isn't Enough

"Cover your mouth when you cough!" is a well-remembered phrase from our childhood and I catch myself wanting to use it today when someone coughs in my face. We all know about covering our mouths, about using our elbows instead of our hands to cover, about washing our hands, and about frequently using hand sanitizers. What many of us don't know about is a more effective preventive measure: nasal washing.

Sneezing is the body's way of clearing dirty and irritated noses. We cringe when someone coughs or sneezes on us. Both the influenza and cold viruses thrive in the nasal environment which has the temperature, humidity and pH they prefer. From the nose, viruses also have a better chance of invading the body's cells. Have you ever noticed how often your friends, family members and colleagues touch their noses? This is why washing hands makes sense. Well, washing the nose makes sense too. It is human nature to touch our noses on the average of three times each hour, and the chance of carrying germs to and from the nose is significant. Clearly, the nose is a primary source of contagious respiratory infections and as such should be cleansed regularly.

Hypertonic saline nasal rinses have been proven to reduce the need for allergy and cold medications, to prevent symptoms related to nasal congestion, and to thin the thick secretions that accompany colds and flu. Just as tooth brushing cleans and refreshes the mouth, nasal rinsing cleans and refreshes the nose. People who include this practice as part of their daily hygiene are getting fewer colds and other respiratory problems; they are noticing the difference in the quality of their lives. They may also be spreading fewer germs to others.

So cover your mouth when you cough, wash your hands frequently, but if you really want to do all you can to prevent colds and flu, wash your nose regularly. Your family, your friends and, most importantly, your nose will thank you for it.

Stacey M. Kerr, MD
Family Physician
Santa Rosa, California

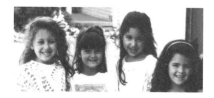

Asthma: Inflammation of the Airways

Asthma is a chronic inflammatory disease that affects your airways, the tubes that carry air in and out of your lungs. If you have asthma, the inside walls of your airways are inflamed, making the airways swollen and sensitive. They tend to react strongly to things that you are allergic to or find irritating. When the airways react, they get narrower, they produce more mucus, and less air flows through to your lung tissue. This causes symptoms like wheezing, coughing, chest tightness and trouble breathing, which tend to be worse at night and in the early morning.

Normal Bronchial Tubes   Asthmatic Bronchial Tubes

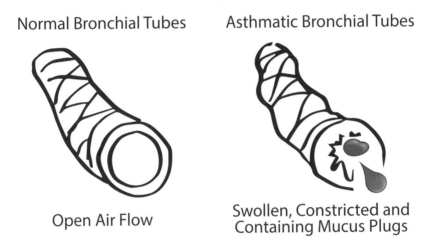

Open Air Flow   Swollen, Constricted and Containing Mucus Plugs

Asthma is one of the leading chronic childhood diseases in the United States and a major cause of childhood disability. Childhood asthma prevalence more than doubled from 1980 to the mid-1990s and remains at historically high levels. The factors driving this pattern are still not fully understood, but we know that contributing factors include increased pollution, processed foods, and in general, unhealthy lifestyles.

The modern medical practitioner helps children and adults with asthma manage their symptoms with inhalers, steroids, nebulizers to vaporize medication into the lungs, and other medications. Too little attention is focused on avoidance of individual triggers and prevention of asthma exacerbations. All patients should have an "Asthma Action Plan" to help them manage their lung disease, and a large part of that plan is avoidance of asthma triggers. Since triggers are a primary cause of asthma exacerbations, it only makes sense to include regular nasal washing as part of an aggressive preventive program. The nose is the filter that protects our lungs. Keep the filter clean, avoid asthma triggers, and you will find you have fewer asthma exacerbations. Prevention is *always* better than treatment!

Some of the more common asthma triggers include exercise, allergens, environmental irritants and viral infections. Families with children who have asthma report that this illness influences a range of decisions concerning home furnishings, carpets, lifestyle, household spending, holidays and pets.

Facts! Asthma Is A Serious And Expensive Health Problem!

- ✓ Asthma costs the United States $56 billion each year.
- ✓ In 2009, the average yearly cost of care for a child with asthma was $1,039.
- ✓ In 2008 there were 10.5 million missed days of school due to asthma.
- ✓ In 2008, there were 14.2 million missed days of work due to asthma.
- ✓ Every day, about nine people die from asthma.
- ✓ In 2010, 18.7 million adults had asthma - that's one in twelve adults.
- ✓ In 2010, 7 million children had asthma - that's one in eleven children.
- ✓ In 2009, 3,388 people died from asthma.

(From the Center for Disease Control
National Asthma Control Program)

Asthma Triggers

✓ Allergens
✓ Animal dander (from the skin, hair, saliva or feathers of animals)
✓ Dust mites
✓ Cockroaches
✓ Pollen from trees, grasses and weeds
✓ Mold
✓ Cigarette smoke
✓ Air pollution
✓ GERD (reflux)
✓ Infection - sinus, throat, chest
✓ Cold air or changes in weather
✓ Strong odors, like those from painting or cooking
✓ Scented products
✓ Strong emotional expression (including crying or laughing hard)
✓ Stress
✓ Medications such as aspirin and beta-blockers
✓ Sulfites in food (dried fruit) or beverages (wine)
✓ Irritants or allergens in the workplace (chemicals, dust, etc...)

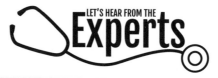

Asthma and the Nose

Asthma is a common childhood and adult ailment, one which all primary care physicians evaluate and treat.

The issue is this: like the nasal area, the bronchial tubes, which connect the upper airway to the lungs, develop congestion with swelling and increased mucus production.

For years, asthma was thought of as a separate condition from allergies. Now we know better. In fact, a majority of asthma cases are directly related to upper airway allergies. Rarely does an asthmatic patient come in complaining of tight chest or coughing without a preceding history of nasal or sinus congestion. This actually is no surprise.

If one breathes through the nose, the air is filtered and warm. If the nose is congested, mouth breathing is required but this bypasses both air filtering and air warming. Thus, unfiltered, cool air aggravates the bronchial tubes, resulting in constriction of the airway muscle, increased airway mucus production and airway "reactivity" or sensitivity.

Yes, there are many medications which treat the symptoms of asthma, and they are effective. There are steroids (inhibit the natural immune response), medications that dilate the bronchial tube muscles (prevent them from constricting) and other chemicals, which affect the immune response to "inflammatory mediators," just to name a few.

In my practice, I approach my patients with asthma as any family physician would. The difference is this: I also evaluate the nose and sinuses. Without addressing these areas, the asthma is only partially treated. In fact, when upper airways are maintained clean and free of irritants, asthma remains quiet.

> *The last thing I wish to offer my patient is another medication, on top of antihistamines, decongestants, bronchodilators, nasal and inhaled steroids and perhaps antibiotics. Therefore, I suggest a good nasal wash to clean the upper airway.*
>
> *Over the years, I have witnessed a reduction of asthma episodes in addition to a reduced dependency on medications when nasal washing is incorporated into a daily habit. Simple and effective.*
>
> George Prica, MD
> Columbia Family Medical Group
> Columbia, Missouri

A Family's Relief

❝ *I have suffered with asthma and allergies since birth and experience recurrent sinus infections. My mother showed me how to wash. Needless to say, the sinus infection cleared up quickly. I am now a devoted user. It definitely helps me deal with all the pollen. My children have started washing daily as well!* **❞**

Linda B., Memphis, Tennessee

Free At Last

❝ *I have diseased sinuses from years of allergy attacks and recurrent sinus infections. I had gotten used to not being able to fully breathe through my nose, and gave up on using nasal sprays and various medications that only treated the symptoms.*

I started washing as soon as I received my kit. It took me about three tries to get the proper angle and flow. The tissues in one of my nostrils were completely swollen, so at first, it was difficult to push the solution through. However, once I had used the system a few times, I noticed a dramatic difference in the condition of my nasal tissues. I was able to actually breathe through my nose almost immediately. Now, I wash my nose every morning and evening, just like brushing my teeth.

This has made such a difference for me that I plan to stop using adhesive strips on my nose when I go to sleep at night. I don't think I will need them anymore! The best part, in my opinion, is that this is a completely natural way to clean the sinuses and nasal membranes, which in turn keeps them healthy, eliminating the need for medications. **99**

Heather R, Hollywood, Florida

Sleep and Breathing Problems — More Serious Than You May Think

 Snoring is a common sleep disorder that can affect people at any age, although it occurs more frequently in men and in people who are overweight. Snoring has a tendency to get worse as a person ages. Close to 45% of adults snore occasionally, while 25% are habitual snorers.

Children need deep restorative sleep, and those who have difficulty breathing while asleep suffer in surprising ways. They may lose their appetite, their ability to learn well, and their growth may be slowed. In other words, they may appear to be normal but actually failing to thrive. I learned this lesson from Lily, a sweet five-year-old girl who was brought to me by her parents after many doctors had tried to figure out why she would not eat and why she was persistently off the low end of the growth charts. After going over her medical history and all the lab tests done so far, I noticed that she was a mouth breather so I asked if she snored. Yes, she did. We evaluated her adenoids which turned out to be abnormally large, and the parents decided to have them removed. It was the difference between night and day! Lily regained her appetite, quit snoring, and within the year was back on the growth charts and growing like a weed. Now I don't usually recommend adenoidectomies, but Lily is a good example of how severely affected children can be if they are simply unable to sleep well.

Snoring occurs when the flow of air through the mouth and nose is physically obstructed, and the walls of the throat vibrate during breathing. This results in the distinctive sounds of snoring. Airflow can be obstructed by conditions which cause narrow nasal airways. During sleep, a person must work harder to breathe because of these partially blocked nasal passages. At times, the soft tissues at the back of the throat collapse and vibrate. Some people snore only during allergy season or when they have a sinus infection. Deformities of the nose such as a deviated septum or nasal polyps, both described later in this chapter, can also cause obstruction and sleep problems.

Nasal washing is an effective way to reduce or eliminate snoring. A college professor I met a few years ago found out just how effective washing can be.

A CPAP machine can help address snoring caused by sleep apnea, but for some people who snore CPAP may not be the answer. A sleep study is the only way to tell. I have seen many who experience snoring and poor sleep quality merely from a stuffy nose. Many CPAP users benefit from washing the nasal passages prior to sleep to ensure open nasal passages. In this situation, a regular routine of nasal washing can make the difference between restful sleep and waking up fatigued.

A Good Night's Sleep for Two

66 *Dr. Hana talked with me about the benefits of nose washing and helping me with my snoring. I tried nose washing and it works! My wife says, 'I don't hear your snoring any more, what have you done?' I told her about the addition to my daily hygiene routine. She was as amazed as I was. I can breathe easier. I think of washing my nose as similar to brushing my teeth.* **99**

Michael S. Smith, PhD, Professor of Teacher Education
Missouri Western State University, St. Joseph, Missouri

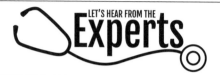

Sleep Apnea and Snoring

Sleep apnea affects more than fifteen million people, with many patients still undiagnosed. In the past a patient snoring during sleep was considered comical. Spouses of patients with sleep apnea would complain that a partner's snoring was disrupting their sleep. The spouse could not sleep because their partner was "holding their breath." Today physicians and health care providers realize that snoring is no joke. Snoring can be a sign of a bigger problem called Obstructive Sleep Apnea. Sleep apnea occurs when tissues in the throat relax during sleep, causing a blockage of the airway. This blockage causes the patient to stop breathing, leading to decreased oxygen levels and disruptions in the patient's sleep cycle. Hypertension, stroke, daytime sleepiness, depression, headaches, forgetfulness, fatigue, memory loss, decreased REM (deep) sleep and diabetes are a few of the proven consequences of untreated sleep apnea.

Snoring, especially when accompanied by episodes of sleep apnea, can be cause for concern and warrants mentioning to your physician, who may send you for a sleep study to evaluate your risk.

Once sleep apnea is diagnosed, a prescription for a CPAP (continuous positive airway pressure) machine is offered as a way to increase airflow to the patient's airway. Keeping a constant respiratory rate alleviates snoring (when caused by sleep apnea) which allows for a more restful and continuous night's sleep. Patients wake feeling rested and alert.

Sinus congestion is one of the leading complaints of CPAP side effects and I have found nasal washing helps by rinsing the nasal passages, decreasing sinus congestion, and allowing air to flow more easily. Something as simple as nasal congestion can derail a patient's efforts to continue therapy. Nasal washing rinses and moisturizes the nasal passages and can help patients be more successful in their CPAP or oxygen therapy. CPAP users can improve their comfort and success rate when nasal washing is incorporated into their daily routine, indirectly decreasing the risk for stroke, hypertension, diabetes or depression. The side effects of untreated sleep apnea are very severe, and nasal washing is one of the most vital tools a respiratory therapist has to treat nasal congestion and dryness caused by CPAP therapy.

Kelly Kilgore-Bietsch
Respiratory Therapist, Columbia, Missouri

Vocal Cord Dysfunction (VCD)

 Most people have never heard of Vocal Cord Dysfunction but as a pediatrician, I see this from time to time. It is not uncommon and certainly a diagnosis to consider when a teenager comes to see me with a complaint of coughing. VCD is often misdiagnosed as either asthma or exercise-induced bronchospasm. As a result, many individuals with VCD are treated inappropriately, unnecessarily exposing them to the potentially harmful side effects of asthma medications.

This condition is typically caused by exercise in adolescents and by environmental irritants in adults. Of course, in a diagnosis of VCD, asthma and underlying conditions need to be ruled out: irritable larynx syndrome, acid reflux, complications from asthma medications, stress or other unknown issues.

Patients with exercise-induced VCD, particularly adolescents, learn to use breathing exercises as a warm-up before sports as a preventive measure. This can involve learning how to breathe efficiently with the focus of the breath more in the front of the mouth versus in the throat. Breathing in through the nose and blowing the air out through the front of the mouth is often accomplished more easily and effectively with regular nasal washing. Breathing exercises used in yoga practice can also assist in alleviating VCD.

Ears and Hearing Problems

The nose is the main influence in sinus and ear infections. We have all experienced the sensation of ear popping or pain when we fly or dive. In order to function properly, and without pain or pressure, the middle ear must be at the same pressure as the external ear. This equalization of pressure occurs via the Eustachian tube which leads from the middle portion of the ear to the back of the throat. When the ears pop while yawning or swallowing or flying, the Eustachian tubes are adjusting the air pressure in the middle ears. An air bubble travels upward in the tube and this is a sign that the tube is not "glued" shut; it is open and mucus is bubbling down and out into the throat. It is vital for the Eustachian tube to remain open if equal pressure is to be maintained on both sides of the eardrum. This cannot be accomplished if there is a mucus plug blocking drainage of the tube or if there is swelling of the opening in the throat which prevents airflow.

For more information about children and ear problems, see "Children and Ears" on page 128 and the section on ears on pages 29–31.

Eustachian Tube Dysfunction (ETD)

The first requirement for a properly functioning ear is to have the Eustachian tubes clear. Eustachian tube dysfunction (ETD) is the most common concern with the ear. This can occur as a result of congestion from any source, including blockage of proper drainage caused by enlarged adenoids or tonsils, or from the inflammation resulting from GERD. Even a sinus infection can cause blockage by mucus plugs blocking the Eustachian tube. The result of ETD can be decreased hearing, dizziness, ringing or even eventual infection.

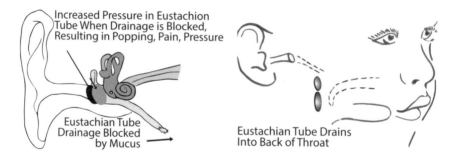

Increased Pressure in Eustachion Tube When Drainage is Blocked, Resulting in Popping, Pain, Pressure

Eustachian Tube Drainage Blocked by Mucus

Eustachian Tube Drains Into Back of Throat

Outer Ear Infection - Swimmers Ear

Swimmers ear has nothing to do with middle ear infections and nothing to do with blockage of the Eustachian tube. This is an infection of the outer ear (ear canal) and most often related to stagnant water residing in the outer ear. This is a set-up for infection in the canal because of the moist warm environment. An infection here requires a dramatic change in the level of acidity in the outer ear to inhibit growth of the infectious colonies. Either antibiotic drops are required, or sometimes a solution can be used which will alter the pH, inhibiting bacteria from growing. This can be tried with 50/50 sterile water/vinegar or hydrogen peroxide mixture. Even a hair dryer can be used to dry out the moisture and inhibit the bacteria's ability to multiply.

Those with recurrent swimmers ear should remember to dry the outer ear canals immediately after swimming or other exposure to water. Because the outer ear does not communicate with the nose, nose washing will not have a direct effect on this type of infection.

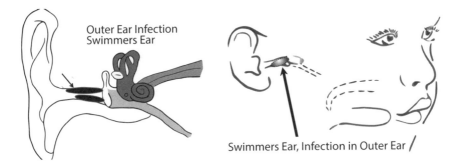

Swimmers Ear, Infection in Outer Ear

Middle Ear Infection (Otitis Media)

I have never examined a child with an inner ear infection who did not experience a preceding stuffy or runny nose. Because of the architecture of a child's Eustachian tube, kids are more prone to ear infections. But one must differentiate an ear infection which requires antibiotics from an ear infection which does not. Many medical doctors will offer antibiotics if the eardrum appears red but we have learned that this is not always necessary, especially if your physician is able to provide close follow-up care. In my experience, a walk-in clinic or emergency room doctor will be more likely to prescribe an antibiotic than a primary physician who knows the family well.

According to the American Academy of Pediatrics (AAP), an infection in the middle ear *(otitis media)* does not necessarily require an antibiotic. The AAP recently warned pediatricians to consider waiting before prescribing antibiotics if possible - that is, if the clinical situation is not too severe. Nasal hygiene, cleaning the opening to the Eustachian tube so that the fluid can drain, is the single most important thing one can do. Of course, if a very young child is experiencing a high fever, or if symptoms persist for an extended period, antibiotics may be required.

When only fluid but no infection is present, the condition is referred to as *serous otitis media*. The fluid often thickens into a glue-like substance if allowed to remain stagnant for weeks or months. In fact, the longer it is present the more difficult it is to encourage normal or natural draining. The glue-like mucus becomes intertwined in those tiny bones *(ossicles)* and aggressive treatment should be considered. If not, hearing loss can develop.

Ear congestion and infections can become very serious and cause permanent hearing loss, a life-changing event. This is why a basic understanding of how the nose and the ears are related is so important. But for one to experience healthy middle ears and Eustachian tubes, a clean nose is vital. Daily washing can go a long way toward relieving and preventing ear problems, including hearing loss.

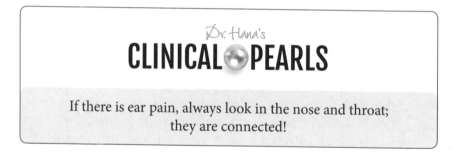

Dr. Hana's
CLINICAL PEARLS

If there is ear pain, always look in the nose and throat;
they are connected!

Bad Breath (Halitosis)

 We all are troubled by bad breath on occasion, but some suffer from this daily. It can be embarrassing to have this problem, despite how aggressively you brush your teeth. The foul odor can result from bacteria on the tongue, the tonsils, the adenoids or from sinus drainage or dehydration. The bacteria that contribute to bad breath are often organisms that live without oxygen *(anaerobic)*. This type of bacteria breaks down and digests proteins in food we eat or in mucus and phlegm, and that process releases odorous sulfur compounds.

This is why people who suffer from infections of the sinuses, ears and throat, from chronic postnasal drip, and from reflux (GERD) are prone to bad breath. This explains why parents of sick and infected children often tell me, "My kid smells sick." I always believe them.

If you still have your tonsils, you may be harboring a pool of bacteria that can result in a complex of mucus and sulfur compounds which love to live in the cracks, crevices and pockets of the tonsils. They're called *tonsilloliths*, or "tonsil stones." Many times, when I have been asked by patients to "See what is stuck in my throat," tonsilloliths is what I find.

What to do about bad breath?

- ✓ Avoid drying agents such as antihistamines.
- ✓ Stay well hydrated; drink plenty of water.
- ✓ Avoid "dry mouth," the most common initiator of bad breath and a great environment for those bacteria to generate sulfur compounds.
- ✓ Address sinus issues, including postnasal drip, with regular nasal washing.

Nose Bleeds (Epistaxis)

 Most of us have experienced the relatively common occurrence of a nosebleed at some time in our lives. The diagnosis is a simple one to make, usually made by the doctor looking into the nose *(direct visualization.)* If the bleeding is from the front portion *(anterior)* of the nose, by far the most common of the two types of nose bleeds, the blood drains out through the nostrils. This bleeding originates from a group of blood vessels called Kiesselbach's area.

The second type of epistaxis is caused by bleeding from the back portion of the nose *(posterior)* and is potentially more likely to require medical attention. This blood usually drains down the back of the throat. Fresh and clotted blood can also flow down into the stomach. This can irritate the stomach, resulting in nausea, vomiting, and exacerbation of the original nosebleed. Although not common, it can be serious.

Kiesselbach's Area

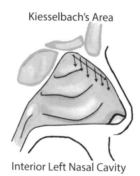

Interior Left Nasal Cavity

Why do some people develop nosebleeds?

The cause of nosebleeds can generally be divided into three categories: local causes, systemic causes (whole body issues), or unknown causes.

Local or common causes:

- ✓ Local trauma (including nose blowing, nose picking, sharp blow to the face)
- ✓ Drying of the nasal mucous membrane (ex: allergies, age, environmental irritation, chemical inhalants, dry air during winter months)

- ✓ Prolonged and improper use of nasal steroid sprays
- ✓ Use of oxygen via a nasal cannula, the device used to deliver extra oxygen through a plastic tube with two prongs placed in the nostrils.
- ✓ Infections: rhinitis, sinusitis, colds
- ✓ Insertion of foreign bodies, usually by children
- ✓ Perforations in the nasal septum
- ✓ Illegal drug use (cocaine or other inhaled substance)
- ✓ Surgery

Systemic or rare causes:

- ✓ Allergies
- ✓ Infections, such as AIDS
- ✓ Arteriosclerosis
- ✓ Benign or malignant tumors in the area of the nose
- ✓ Bleeding and clotting disorders (e.g., thrombocytopenia, liver disease, coagulopathies, and anticoagulant use)
- ✓ Medication side effects: aspirin, antihistamine, warfarin, ibuprofen, isotretinoin (Retin-a), desmopressin and others
- ✓ Blood abnormalities, including malignancies
- ✓ Poorly controlled high blood pressure
- ✓ Pregnancy
- ✓ Alcohol (due to dilation of blood vessels)

Treatment

The flow of blood normally stops when the blood clots, that is, when the blood forms a plug. This process takes time. Applying direct pressure by pinching the soft fleshy part of the nose can stop the flow and allow clotting to occur. Pressure should be firm and be applied for at least ten minutes *without releasing pressure even for a second - set a timer! Don't let up even to change hands!* It is also important to keep the head in the neutral position; do not lean the head back because this makes the blood drain down the throat and can cause complications. Spit out any blood that flows into the mouth; do not swallow it. Do not pack the nose with tissues or gauze. There is no benefit to pinching the bridge of the nose.

In the past, it was routine to recommend the application of cold such as an ice pack to the forehead or sucking on an ice cube to stop bleeding from the nose. It was believed the exposure to cold would promote constriction of local blood vessels, thus slow down the bleeding. However, we now know that these practices do not have any significant effect on slowing or stopping nosebleeds.

If you have applied pressure for a full ten minutes and the nose is still bleeding, contact your physician. There are medications that can be used directly on the bleeding area if necessary. Direct chemical cautery (using silver nitrate) of any bleeding vessels or professional packing of the nose with ribbon gauze or an absorbent dressing may be necessary to stop the bleeding. Ongoing bleeding despite good nasal packing is a surgical emergency.

Recurrent epistaxis resulting from a dry nasal mucosa is reduced by saline nasal washings two to three times per day, lubricating the nose with ointment or creams like Vaseline or antibiotic ointment, and installing a humidifier in the bedroom.

Nosebleeds are rarely dangerous unless the bleeding is prolonged and heavy. The elderly and those with co-existing illnesses, particularly those with illnesses and medications that affect blood clotting, should be closely monitored.

Nasal Polyps

Polyps are growths of tissue, often in response to chronic irritation or inflammation. Imagine finger-like tissue projections that can plug up the waterworks. They block passages and prevent normal drainage and normal breathing. You may have a single soft jelly-like nasal polyp or several clustered together like grapes. They are difficult to live with and even more difficult to treat.

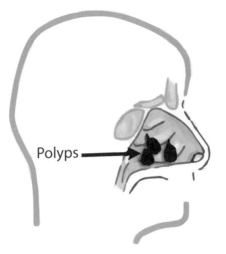

Polyps

Risk factors include:

- ✓ Asthma
- ✓ Chronic allergies
- ✓ Chronic sinus infections
- ✓ Sensitivity to aspirin or non-steroidal anti-inflammatory drugs like ibuprofen
- ✓ Age; more common in people older than 40
- ✓ Fungal sinusitis
- ✓ Family/genetic predisposition
- ✓ Cystic Fibrosis

Symptoms that may indicate the presence of nasal polyps

- ✓ Mouth breathing
- ✓ A chronic runny nose
- ✓ Persistent stuffiness
- ✓ Recurrent or chronic sinus infections
- ✓ Loss or diminishment of your sense of smell
- ✓ Dull headaches
- ✓ Snoring and sleep apnea

How Nasal Polyps Develop

Nasal polyps can develop in the mucous membranes lining your nose or sinus cavities. Polyps are the product of ongoing inflammation which causes the blood vessels in the lining of your nose and sinuses to become more permeable, allowing water to accumulate in the cells. Simply put, the tissue swells and over time, as gravity pulls on these waterlogged tissues, polyps develop.

To help diagnose nasal polyps, the doctor will take a detailed medical history and will examine your nose with a *nasopharyngeal scope*, a small lighted camera that allows direct visualization. You may even get a computerized tomography (CT) scan to help determine the size and exact location of the polyps, including any polyps in your sinuses.

A small single polyp may never be an issue, but large or multiple polyps block the air flow through the nose and result in congestion and infections. These small growths often develop in the osteomeatal complex and due to their location, can cause obstructive sleep apnea, asthma exacerbations, and infections. Note: If your child is diagnosed with nasal polyps, screening for Cystic Fibrosis should be part of the evaluation.

When your doctor finds polyps, there are medications that can help - topical or systemic steroids, antihistamines, perhaps antibiotics. But we know that steroids are not your friend for long-term use. Sometimes the polyps will be removed surgically but even this treatment is not permanent or complete. The roots of these growths are like tree roots - very deep - so they often grow back.

The best long-term plan for managing nasal polyps addresses the cause first: chronic inflammation of the nasal mucosa. Washing the nose several times a day is effective in decreasing the inflammatory reaction that leads to polyp formation, if the wash is with hypertonic buffered solution. This not only helps keep polyps small and less obstructive, but may prevent the development of new growth, perhaps completely avoiding the need for surgery.

Deviated Nasal Septum

 The nasal septum is the wall, the midline cartilage of the nose that separates the two airways and the nostrils. A deviated septum is present when there is a shift from the midline or center position. These deviations can occur from genetics, normal growth variants or trauma (broken nose, fall, surgery).

Minor deviations are common and usually do not cause symptoms or require any treatment. If, however, the midline cartilage is deviated significantly, the opposite turbinates may swell over time to fill the resulting empty space. This swelling is referred to as *compensatory hypertrophy*, and may cause more problems than the actual deviated septum! The resulting airflow obstruction increases the risk of infections, headaches, increased allergy symptoms, and even nose bleeds.

If the deviation is minor, persistent nose washing will reduce any symptoms. If surgery is required to reconstruct and reposition the septal cartilage, one should wash prior to surgery to shrink any swelling and offer the surgeon healthy tissues to work with.

When washing with a deviated septum, or any cause of obstruction on one side, always begin on the congested side first. If you are successful in having the solution exit the opposite side, then you can feel safe in flushing through the uncongested side as well. If you are not able to flush through the congested side, do not force. I repeat: DO NOT FORCE. Continue to wash gently with a hypertonic solution, multiple times, on the congested side only, until you succeed. Refer to the section on congestion on page 108 for specific instructions.

Check with your doctor if you are unsuccessful after a few days of trying. If the solution is forced through with too much pressure, you can damage an eardrum!

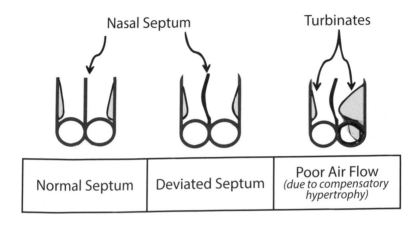

Normal Septum	Deviated Septum	Poor Air Flow *(due to compensatory hypertrophy)*

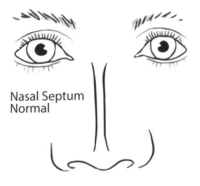

Nasal Septum Normal

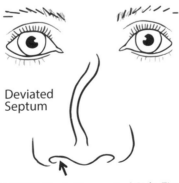

Deviated Septum

ALWAYS Flush Congested Side First

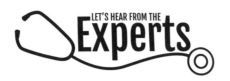

LET'S HEAR FROM THE

The Almost Perfect Nose

As a nurse practitioner who has treated thousands of allergy fighters in a Midwest sinus and allergy clinic in the heart of allergy country, I talk to patients a lot about their noses. Most of our patients who are daily users of nasal saline wash are healthier; they come to see me less often. They are able to breathe better by rinsing out dust, pollens or viruses before those pollutants settle in their nasal tissue.

Most of us do not have a perfect nose, like those with a deviated septum. This narrowing of one side of the nasal passage can limit our breathing, especially important at night. I have found that a simple nose wash can make all the difference, allowing the air to pass through the nose, rather than through the mouth. Rinsing out irritants and decongesting one's nose with a saline wash may also improve sleep…for you and your family.

Jane M. Cooper, RN, BC, FNP
Columbia, Missouri

Decreased or Absence of Smell (*Anosmia*) and Taste (*Ageusia*)

Anosmia is an absence of the ability to smell. *Ageusia* is an absence of the ability to taste. These two important senses are forever linked; if we lose our ability to smell, we also lose most of our ability to taste.

When you chew food, chemicals are released that trigger receptors in the upper reaches of your nose. These receptors then trigger the brain to create the sensation of taste. If those chemicals cannot get to the nasal receptors, the brain cannot give us information about taste. So when the nose is compromised by inflammation, allergies, polyps, or from excess mucus, our ability to taste is also affected. Anyone who has had a cold or sinus infection has experienced the anosmia and ageusia that goes with a stuffy nose.

Smell is a sense we take for granted, only appreciating how important it is when it is taken away. People with anosmia have real problems with safety issues, eating, and feelings of insecurity because they cannot detect hazards like leaking gas, smoke, pollutants, spoiled foods, or even their own body odor. Changes in the sense of smell can weaken our immune system and even contribute to digestive disorders.

Memories, moods, and our general sense of well-being are more dependent on our ability to smell than we may realize. It is no surprise that some who lose this underappreciated sense will struggle with depression directly related to their anosmia.

Damage to the olfactory system affects 1-2% of Americans. Most of these people are over the age of 65 since some loss is a normal part of aging. And taste? Most individuals start life with about 10,000 taste buds that replace themselves every two weeks. But older people may only have *half* that many taste buds - even less if they smoke cigarettes. Aging of both the nose and our taste buds can create real problems for the elderly. I once knew a patient who lost his sense of taste and smell and was eating sour cream for weeks, thinking it was yogurt!

Regular nasal washing, by preventing congestion, can maintain access to the olfactory receptors in the nose. It's the first-line treatment for anosmia and ageusia. But nasal woes and aging are not the only culprits. Head trauma, surgical scarring, nonmalignant tumors, and occupational exposure to chemicals can contribute to the loss. Some of these causes are quite treatable, so if anosmia is persistent it is advised that you see your doctor.

Common Causes of Anosmia:

- Normal aging
- Recent upper respiratory Infection
- Runny Nose
- Stuffy Nose
- Common Cold
- Allergies
- Foreign Body in the Nose
- Sinusitis
- Nasal Polyps
- Smoking
- Exposure to Toxic Chemicals
- Use of Nasal Decongestants

A Loyal Nasal Washer

❝ *I was too congested to create a flow from one nostril to the other; nasal washing really helped me blow more out than I could before. I know the importance of keeping the nasal passages clean. I'd almost completely lost my ability to smell or taste due to prolonged nasal congestion and sinus irritation over many years, but I noticed these senses coming back to me a few weeks after starting a regular routine of washing twice each day.* **❞**

Cory P., Miami, Florida

Taste of Food Returns

❝ *My husband and I sat next to Dr. Hana on a flight to St. Louis. We decided to try a nose wash since my husband has difficulty with his sinuses and tends to lose his sense of taste. Along with a nebulizer he uses daily, the two seem to be the right combination and I no longer have to describe the taste of his food to him or whether or not a particular flower is fragrant!* **❞**

Lynn N, Long Island, New York

Immotile Cilia

 Immotile Cilia Syndrome, or Primary Ciliary Dyskinesia (PCD), describes an inherited condition in which the cilia fail to beat normally. This means the cilia cannot clear mucus out of the respiratory passages resulting in mucus becoming stuck and eventually blocking the airways. Mucus is an excellent breeding ground for bacteria and when it remains in place for extended periods, it may become infected. The bacteria release chemicals that can damage tissues in the area, especially in the lungs. In addition, the body produces special cells in response to irritants referred to as *inflammatory cells*. These cells can release chemicals such as enzymes, which cause further local tissue damage. People with Immotile Cilia Syndrome suffer frequent infections of the lungs, ears, throat and sinuses. Unless treated, this may lead to permanent damage.

Nasal washing does what immotile cilia do not; it clears mucus from the nasal passages, allowing unobstructed airflow and eliminating an environment in which harmful bacterial can cause infection. Keeping the nasal airways clear helps protect the rest of the respiratory tract, especially when cilia are unable to perform their vital function.

Cystic Fibrosis

 According to data collected by the Cystic Fibrosis (CF) Foundation, about 30,000 Americans, 3,000 Canadians and 20,000 Europeans have Cystic Fibrosis. About 2,500 babies are born with CF each year in the United States. This inherited chronic disease affects the lungs and digestive system. There is involvement of the sinuses, with or without nasal polyps. The abnormal gene results in the production of unusually thick, sticky mucus that blocks the lungs, leading to life-threatening lung infections. There is also obstruction of the pancreatic ducts, which prevents natural enzymes from helping the body break down and absorb food.

Patients with CF can develop a variety of symptoms, including:

- ✓ Persistent coughing, at times with phlegm
- ✓ Wheezing or shortness of breath
- ✓ Poor growth and weight loss in spite of a good appetite
- ✓ Frequent lung infections
- ✓ Nasal polyps leading to chronic sinus infections

Living with Cystic Fibrosis often entails taking multiple medications and physical therapy. Although the first treatment plan for CF includes medications, surgery has been heavily relied upon for extensive sinus, polyps and nasal issues. Due to the high recurrence rate, repeated surgeries can be required. Nasal hypertonic saline rinses have been found to improve both sinus and lung function in patients with CF, simply by increasing airway hydration and improving mucus clearance. Over the years I have personally seen how hypertonic nasal irrigation used daily can really make a significant improvement in the quality of life and the number of infections and complications that these patients experience.

Cystic Fibrosis Means Nose Washing is a Life Saver

66 *My son Ashford is eight years old. He is a beautiful, tremendously smart, amazing little boy! Ashford loves to make people laugh and has the biggest heart I know. Ashford also has Cystic Fibrosis. We received the diagnosis while I was pregnant. He was the fifth in utero diagnosis in Georgia. This enabled us a great advantage. We were able to meet all of Ashford's doctors, and learn about CF before he was even born. We felt very blessed to be ahead of the game. Ashford has been on pancreatic enzymes since he was three days old. In a day he takes about 20 different pills and does five different nebulizer treatments, more when he is sick. He does this along with two different 30-minute vest sessions to help thin out and remove the extra mucus in his lungs.*

We have been able to take preventative measures from the very beginning, in our fight against CF. While we cannot prevent everything, it has definitely made a difference in his quality of life.

He stayed very well until he was four years old when he had his first major lung infection and hospital stay. His lungs cleared but he was still having other issues such as puffy cheeks, mouth breathing and snoring. Ashford's wonderful ENT diagnosed Ashford with significant sinus disease, filled with polyps. Ashford underwent two sinus surgeries to remove troublesome polyps.

Ashford's doctors suggested that we start nasal washing. I was all for it, because it was natural and not adding one more medicine to his little body. The doctors explained that nasal washing would help clean out extra mucus as well as any irritants and bacteria. Ashford was only four when he started the nasal washing. He was willing to try because he hoped it would help keep him from having any more surgeries.

We tried the premixed saline spray, but he did not like how it would rundown the back of his throat. We tried the neti pot and it was too big and awkward for him to do by himself. Plus it did not seem to wash and dry easily. I then searched on the internet for something out there easy enough for kids to do. I found Nasopure. I loved that there were examples of children doing it themselves, as well as testimonials.

Ashford took to washing very easily and was amazed at how it made him feel. He said 'This feels so good, can I do it again right now!' He does the washing twice a day, no matter what when he is well. CF produces thick mucus so there are times when he is sick that nasal washing was the only thing that would unclog his nose. He will come and ask for it. One day we did it a twelve times in a 24-hour period. There is nothing like watching your child struggling to breathe. It is a great comfort to know that something so easy and so natural can bring such relief.

It has been three years since Ashford's last sinus surgery. He has not had one sinus infection. He is still on all of his Cystic Fibrosis medicines and treatments. Ashford is very compliant regarding all of his treatments including his nasal washing. He did have a hospital stay six months ago, but it was due to a CF lung infection.

Nasal washing will go along with his daily CF treatments for the rest of his life. It is definitely something that works and helps Ashford. While we know that nasal washing will not cure CF or prevent every polyp, we know that it will be one of our weapons as continue to fight to give Ashford a long healthy life.

The Cystic Fibrosis team shares Ashford's story to whoever may be hesitant about nasal washing. **99**

MeLissa G, Villa Rica, Georgia

Better Than Antibiotics...Better Than a Hospital Stay

66 *My son just turned six. He has been on Nasopure for a little over a year right after his first set of sinus surgeries. He also has significant sinus disease due to CF. We needed something to cleanse the sinuses daily and this is perfect. He is a pro at using it. He is on enough meds that I did want something natural. He has told his ENT and allergist and there are now several other kids of all ages at his clinic who use Nasopure! I can firmly attest that he would have had many more sinus infections without it. We use it at least twice a day and if he is having problems with stuffy nose and such we do the rinse several times a day. He always says this is much better than an antibiotic or hospital stay.* **99**

Lisa G, Annandale, Virginia

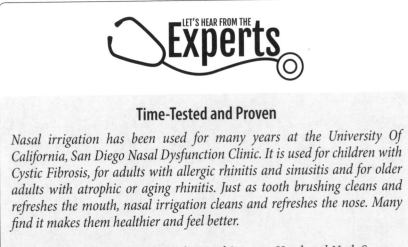

LET'S HEAR FROM THE
Experts

Time-Tested and Proven

Nasal irrigation has been used for many years at the University Of California, San Diego Nasal Dysfunction Clinic. It is used for children with Cystic Fibrosis, for adults with allergic rhinitis and sinusitis and for older adults with atrophic or aging rhinitis. Just as tooth brushing cleans and refreshes the mouth, nasal irrigation cleans and refreshes the nose. Many find it makes them healthier and feel better.

Terence M. Davidson M.D., Professor of Surgery, Head and Neck Surgery, University of California, San Diego, School of Medicine, VA San Diego Health Care System

Resistant Bacteria

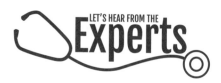

Millions of diverse bacteria coexist peacefully in and on our body; they perform essential nutritive and protective tasks for us. The ones that live in normal and healthy sinuses either crowd out or kill off dangerous bacteria (pathogens) such as Staphylococcus Aureus (SA). Twenty percent of the population carries pathogens without any signs of illness, but they can still unwittingly spread these bacteria to others who may be more susceptible.

Superbug (virulent) strains of SA are among our most feared bacteria; they can release grave and sometimes deadly toxins. Worrisome is the fact that SA has been able to develop a resistance against our most powerful weapon: antibiotics. This is referred to as Methicillin Resistant Staphylococcal Aureus (MRSA). Although MRSA was originally found mainly in hospitals, our communities are now becoming infected. And while there are additional bacteria which are resistant, MRSA is most well-known, with the most exposure in the press.

The risk of resistance developing to SA or MRSA is greatest when treatment relies solely on antibiotics. We treat skin abscesses with antibiotics as well as opening the wound to allow drainage of the infection. This drainage is vital, much like sinus drainage when addressing infections.

When antibiotics are used to treat sinus infections, they do three things. First, they kill off pathogens (potentially harmful bacterial) sensitive to the antibiotic. Second, they also kill off the normal flora. Third, any pathogens that are resistant to the antibiotic now have a chance to overgrow and become a super-infection.

Extinction of normal flora would seriously endanger our health. Maintenance of a healthy balance of microbes is as important as destroying pathogens like SA and MRSA. Health professionals historically have been taught about the "germs" but tend to ignore the dangers of removing the beneficial and normal balance of microbes (flora).

Too often sinus infections become chronic as each antibiotic causes yet another resistant strain to over-grow. The versatility and utility of nasal washing has been overlooked far too long. Nasal washing has the potential to lower SA and MRSA pathogens below toxic levels. The adage "an ounce of prevention is worth a ton of cure," applies perfectly for SA and MRSA infections. Improving hygienic methods both for hospital workers and patients, protecting our normal flora by avoiding exposure to needless antibiotics, as well as draining those infected sinuses with hypertonic buffered saline nose washes will begin to address this worrisome situation.

Marilyn James-Kracke, PhD
Associate Professor
Medical Pharmacology and Physiology
University of Missouri-Columbia

Chapter 12

Normal Life Needs

Can't I Just Buy an Air Filter?

 Air purifiers vary widely in regards to how effectively they remove air pollutants inside the home; some may improve indoor air quality. All air purifiers have some limitations so keep in mind:

- ✓ No air purifier can remove 100% of the pollutants from the air.
- ✓ The most common air purifiers are designed to remove only particles; they have no effect on odors caused by smoke gases.
- ✓ The use of ultraviolet (UV) light in air purifiers does not remove smoke from the air.

Clean Air

❝ *If the air is poor and hazardous to your health and the air filter only works partially, and a mask is only a partial answer, another piece of the 'protective puzzle' may be washing the body's filter.*

I have really horrible allergies that I tried to ignore for many years. I'd pop an antihistamine when I absolutely had to, and just carry tissues everywhere I went. Then I started getting sinus infections that would not stay away; it seemed I was on antibiotics all the time. I was losing time at work and had no energy to do the fun stuff I liked to do on weekends. This was serious! I went to the allergist and started allergy shots. I talked to my ENT doctor and got very few answers other than another prescription. So I started looking at the air I breathe.

I put an ionizer next to my bed so the air would be filtered while I slept. I made sure I washed my sheets in really hot water so the dust mites would be destroyed. I added a huge HEPA filter to my central heating system and immediately felt the difference. My house did not feel toxic to me anymore.

But this didn't fix my problems when I went outside…and I was not about to give up my outdoor fun! So I started washing my nose every single morning, every single evening, and every time I'd come back in from playing outdoors. I hike, I garden, and I ride a motorcycle. That's a lot of exposure.

The nasal washes made the difference. They allow me to leave the safety of my clean home and enjoy the world outside without getting allergy attacks or infections. Since starting daily washes, I have not had to be on antibiotics once.

I'm so grateful. A house air filter and the means to keep my own personal filter clean have made all the difference in my quality of life. **99**

Marie M., Sacramento, California

Industrial Communities

66 *The community where I live is a highly industrial town with two large industries that make a lot of chemicals. At the same time, we are very rural and heavily exposed to insecticides, fertilizers, herbicides, pesticides and farm dust. Spring fever and hay fever are significant problems. Global warming is noticeably increasing the number of allergies that we deal with. Nasal washing is clearly better than saline nasal spray and lot safer than steroid nasal sprays or prescription antihistamines.* **99**

Joseph B., Springfield, Illinois

Professional Voices

 If your voice is the most important instrument in the toolbox you use to make your living, a scratchy throat and stuffy nose isn't just annoying; it's a disaster. Postnasal drip or sinusitis can ruin your day. Singers, announcers, and TV / radio personalities need be able to sing, speak and hear at optimal levels in order to perform well.

Many voice professionals require daily use of allergy medications or nasal steroids. These medications can be expensive, come with unwanted side effects and still only treat the symptoms, not the cause. Nasal washing addresses the source of the problem and actually improves voice quality.

Singers, radio hosts and others who regularly wash their nose tell me that washing is helpful in several ways. The moisturizing effect on the vocal cords prevents drying of membranes and reduces "cracking" of the voice. Singers who wash their nose on a regular basis require less lubrication (drinks) during performances. Those who sing *acapella* especially appreciate the fact that washing opens up the middle ear canal, allowing better capability for subtle changes in tone and pitch.

Underlying asthma, sore throat and allergies may aggravate vocal problems. Stress and overuse can contribute to the development of vocal cord nodules, polyps, chronic laryngitis and hoarseness. Nasal discharge is reduced with regular washings and thus breathing is improved. When a singer or speaker can inhale through the nose without difficulty, the soft palate lifts, creating more space and improving voice quality. Washing may not be the final word in voice health but it is a very important step.

A Singer Sounds Off

66 *As an actor and singer, my body and my voice are also my instrument. Just as I would care for a clarinet or violin, I care for my body and voice on a daily basis. Nose washing regularly allows me to make a daily habit of clearing my sinuses and nasal passages, reducing the frequency of sinus infections, obliterating post-nasal drip, and leaving my head and nose*

feeling clean, clear, and free of pressure. I rinse my nose every day in the shower, eliminating any mess or cleanup, and I keep a container of the saline mix by my sink for easy access. My daily ritual reminds me that I can stay healthy and be ready for the day despite the allergens, pathogens, and other junk that hit me all day. 99

Ryan M, Columbia, Missouri

Radio Host Sounds Clear

66 *I have been using a nose washing system for two years and I swear by it, and after reading Dr. Solomon's book I now know why it works.* 99

Bill Wax, Washington DC
Program Director and Show Host
Sirius/XM Satellite Radio's B.B. King's Bluesville

Good News

66 *I am a morning news anchor for a local television station in Kansas City, Missouri. Not only do I have to deal with early morning hours and an old musty studio, but I also have allergies, which can be disastrous when trying to deliver the news. I had Dr. Hana on as an interview guest and we talked about nasal irrigation and Nasopure. She gave me a bottle and told me to give it a try. Within three days, the puffiness in my eyes went down, my allergies subsided and the actual quality of my voice improved! My voice didn't crack and the tone of my voice actually got a bit deeper and much less nasal! I can certainly tell if I haven't used nasal irrigation for a couple of days based on my on-air voice performance.* 99

Laura Thornquist Fox Morning News Anchor Kansas City, Missouri

Essential for This Traveling Musician

❝ *I am a full-time touring musician who spends 80% of the year on the road. I never leave home without my Nasopure tucked into my toiletries bag. As a traveler, I am constantly in a new environment - sleeping on mysterious couches, hanging out in funky greenrooms, traversing across seasons (sometimes I hit the pollen explosion of spring several times over the course of a month). All these changes can trigger the allergies and asthma I've had since I was a child. I've found that my best defense is a daily nasal rinse with Nasopure. I used to constantly turn to antibiotics to beat off infections, but now that I use Nasopure on a daily basis, I haven't needed antibiotics but once in the last ten years. I traverse the U.S., Canada, and Europe with the travel-size Nasopure, which is super light, takes up very little room, and is good as a preventative measure and a first response to nasal congestion. I'm forever grateful to Dr. Hana for introducing me to Nasopure.* **❞**

David Wax, The David Wax Museum

An Inspired Instrument of Relief

❝ *How do I love my Nasopure? Let me count the ways...*

I was a long time neti pot user for allergies/sinus/cold issues. But after a head and neck injury I was in urgent need of something less stressful on my neck. I found Nasopure after an internet search and was encouraged by the video presentation showing that a young child could so easily use it. I ordered my first Nasopure immediately and was thrilled I could do nasal washing without harm or pain to my neck.

My world changed in 2010 after a dental implant surgery that went terribly wrong and resulted in crushed sinus and an abnormal gaping hole between my sinus and mouth! Regular laser treatments have helped close this hole.

Without prayer, without persistence, without Nasopure I could never have gotten through this.

I continue my career as a professional opera singer and public speaker. I travel with Nasopure at all times and have used it in dressing rooms, on airplane bathrooms, hotels and backstage at the theaters. I recommend it to all my students, singer colleagues, and those who suffer with allergies. Thank you to Dr. Hana for creating this inspired instrument of relief! **99**

Hallie Neill, www.DivaBaritone.com

My Joy of Singing Has Returned

66 *I was a mess. Take it from me, a musician, that a plugged nose and ears was a deterrent from enjoying singing, not to mention hearing it. My ability to function successfully, not only in music, but simple daily living, was being undermined. From my first nasal wash, Dr. Hana's book and techniques made a difference. As the many nasal issues I was able to start enjoying music again. Singing became fun again, I wasn't just doing it because I had too. On the average, I use a hypertonic rinse once in the morning and once in the evening, and have not missed a nasal washing day since. Sure enough, about two or three months after I began nasal washing, not only was I able to function again, but I was also free of my daily antihistamine / decongestant medicines.* **99**

Grady Pope, Cambria, California

Singing Is Easy

❝ *Kindermusik teachers often work with 120 young children a week, and colds are a big problem for teachers… especially singing teachers! Mine last too long and tend to settle in the chest and stay there with mucus discharge and coughing for several weeks. My husband and I really love the nasal washing system. We have both noticed much clearer nasal passages and when we get any hint of a pre-cold feeling, we use nasal washing and we have not developed any colds this season. We sing a lot during the holidays, so this was a real boon to feel well throughout. We have not had a cold this winter season, and the clear feeling in the nostrils is great when we sing. We are both vocal/choral musicians.* **❞**

Virginia C, Modesto, California

 ## Military

American Soldiers in Iraq Have Clean Noses

❝ *I just wanted to let you know that my husband passed out the free nasal washing kits you sent to Iraq and the guys absolutely loved them. It is extremely dusty over there and my husband said they really help.* **❞**

Sheila L., Summertown, Tennessee

Travelers

Already in this book I have pointed out how often people get sick after traveling by air. We put ourselves at risk by spending hours in very close quarters with more than a hundred other people, breathing re-circulated air in small spaces for hours at a time, and touching surfaces teeming with more germs than any of us want to think about.

Whether you are a traveler or work in the travel industry, nasal washing can go a long way toward keeping your body's filter clean and working properly to protect you. Washing your nose helps you stay clear of whatever illnesses passengers bring onto the plane or train, especially helpful if you wash your personal filter immediately after exposure. You may even stay healthy enough to enjoy your time off.

Traveling

66 I wanted to let you know that I took my nasal wash with me to Australia and used it on the fourteen-hour plane ride back and forth from Los Angeles to Sydney to keep my nasal passages moist. It worked very well and I intend to do it again when I go to Thailand in February. 99

Robert Hodge, MD
University of Missouri
Columbia, Missouri

Airplane Virus Knocked Right Out

66 Hi Dr. Hana, I just got back from Australia to Reno, NV. In spite of business class flight I contracted a nasty airplane virus. With my Nasopure I've pretty much completely knocked it out in three days. I wish I had taken it on the plane with me because I may have avoided getting it in the first place or zapped it even sooner. At any rate, the PA in Urgent Care told me to make sure I keep using my Nasopure as it would help me to avoid further complications. As I am a cardiac patient this is especially important. **99**

JoAnn D, Reno, Nevada

Excessive Mucus

66 *I taught my husband how to wash for his travels to India. You don't want to see the stuff that comes out of his nose at the end of a full day out and about in the streets of India! We both recently had a cold, and the nasal irrigation helped a lot in clearing our sinuses.* **99**

Rachel A., New York City, New York

Speak Up

66 *I frequently have to travel for speaking engagements and I have a long history of upper respiratory infections and sinus problems. Several years ago I started taking hand sanitizer with me on flights and wiping down my chair arms and tray table before using it on my own hands. I'd use the hand cleaner every couple of hours; it gave me something to do and I figured it couldn't hurt to try to stay healthy. At the same time I increased the amount of water I was drinking while traveling - trying to stay hydrated and healthy. Those two changes made a big difference in the number of colds I caught after traveling.*

But I still had occasional sinus pain when the plane would descend. The pain was like no other - like hot knives sticking into my forehead - excruciating. So I started taking a decongestant before I'd fly.

Then I found a convenient nasal wash. What a difference!

Now I carry my hand cleaner, use it on my seat and tray table and my hands, and I wash my nose as soon as I get to my hotel room.

I haven't been sick after a trip in over three years. I feel so empowered! **"**

Dr. Kay, San Francisco, California

Smokers

Here's another reason to quit smoking: smoking damages the cilia, those tiny hairs that sweep pollutants out of the nose and lungs and protect against infections. Smokers also lose the ability to appreciate odors and flavors.

Smokers can give their cilia more of a fighting chance against infection and improve their appreciation of the fragrances around them by washing the nose every single day. Washing that is more frequent would be better, but a daily wash should be the minimum.

Let me make this perfectly clear; nasal washing is *not* something you should do instead of quitting smoking; it's something you should do while you smoke, something you should do while you are quitting, and something you should continue to do after you've quit.

Living and Working in Polluted Environments

Many of the people who work in polluted environments earn their living in places we think of as the great outdoors. But that outdoor air isn't always clean and fresh. This is a fact that farmers, ranchers, construction workers, painters and woodworkers know all too well.

People in many areas of construction are subjected to a high volume of airborne pollutants, including chemicals in airborne droplets or fumes, various forms of dust, particles from building materials, fiberglass, etc.

At some job sites workers wear filter masks, but those masks don't catch everything and they can block workers' vision. When that happens, the mask is often discarded. At the end of the day workers' noses and sinuses are filled with the gunk they've been breathing all day.

Even painters who wear expensive and sophisticated filtering masks know that the filter just can't catch all the overspray that is a part of painting; and nose blowing doesn't clear out everything that gets past the mask. Daily nasal washing mitigates long-term risks as well as cleaning out the buildup of the chemicals that make up paints, stains and sealants.

Transit workers and tollbooth collectors are a particularly vulnerable group. Working around automotive air pollution and collecting fares and tolls from hundreds of people every day makes these workers highly vulnerable to whatever illnesses are going around, whatever the season. The constant exposure to automotive exhaust and fumes, and the endless contact with money and the public carry significant risks. Nasal washing can reduce the number of days these workers go to work feeling lousy, or feeling so lousy that they can't go to work.

The work environment is even more challenging for firefighters, who can be surrounded by deadly smoke, fumes, and toxic burning chemicals.

Exposure to smoke is associated with increased symptoms: nose, eyes and throat irritations, coughs, bronchitis, wheezing and asthma attacks. Few professionals would benefit more from nasal washing than those who fight fires.

"Wood dust is an irritant and is carcinogenic to the nasal mucosa. It inhibits its own clearance from the nose." In a study published in the journal *Occupational Medicine* in 1999, researchers gave 46 woodworkers instructions in nasal washing to see if it would reduce nasal symptoms. Not only did the whole group report significantly decreased symptoms, half of them continued the practice on their own voluntarily after one year. They liked the feeling of a clean nose enough to make it part of their daily hygiene.

Stubborn Welder Now Nose Washer

66 *Over the years my brother-in-law has suffered with frequent colds, sinus congestion and bronchitis. He is a welder, and although he now is in a supervisory role, the atmosphere at work is still full of irritants. This winter he has not had a cold, and my sister says he thinks the nasal washing really helps.* 99

Glenda K., Joplin, Missouri

Free To Work

66 *I have been using a saline wash for the nose, twice a day for two years. This has decreased the number of sinus infections I have had to deal with (only two so far this school year) and allowed me to continue working. I had been afraid that the mold in my school would send me into early retirement; now I should be able to finish the year. I have one bottle at home and keep a spare in my suitcase so I won't forget it when I travel. It has helped so much in keeping me healthy and off antibiotics. I have told many people including my neighbor downstairs, who works in a welding shop, a very dirty environment.* 99

Mary G., St Peters, Missouri

Wood Working

66 *The concept of using pressure instead of gravity to clean up my nose just made sense to me. I owned a wood working business for twelve years and had a hell of a time with allergies. I had to take a bunch of medicine to get by and you won't believe the amount of money that I had to spend a month.*

The allergy medicine made me drowsy. One day I had enough. I did some research on the web, and what a surprise when I tried nose washing! My allergies are gone, I can finally breathe better. I also got rid of the drowsiness and most importantly the insane medical bill. I am happy to tell you that I'm off the allergy medication for about five months now and couldn't be happier. Keep up the good work! 🙶

Paco G., McAllen, Texas

Athletes and Sports Enthusiasts

 By now you know that nasal cleanliness is central to good health. It is essential to have a good supply of oxygen if your performance is going to be your best, especially during athletic activities. If the nose is congested, or the airflow is obstructed, the body is not going to perform as well as it could.

Athletes need to perform at their physical peak, yet they hesitate to use medications. The first step to increase athletic performance is as simple as washing the nose, the body's air filter. Nasal washing is particularly useful for anyone encountering air pollutants during their workouts.

Nasal washing works for any athlete at any level of competition: from the weekend players at the public tennis courts, to the world-class pro at Wimbledon, from the guys at the company softball game to professionals playing in the World Series, from the lunchtime hoops crowd at the YMCA to the players in the NBA, from the family reunion flag football contest to the NFL pros. A professional athlete will never fail a drug test by washing their nose, not matter how often he or she washes.

Bicycles and Motorcycles

Active Bicyclist

❝ *I have allergies and asthma but I am a very active bicyclist. We usually ride for 40-50 miles at a clip and, of course, I am breathing in tons of allergens. I have had multitudes of sinus infections and I'm sick of it. A friend of mine was telling me about nasal washing, and I love it. I had never heard of washing my nose or sinuses! I know I will avoid ever having a sinus infection again. My plan is to use the nasal washing system at least once per day and especially after a bike ride.* **❞**

Paul L, Pittsburgh, Pennsylvania

Motorcycle Passion

❝ *I ride a Harley as often as possible - it's my therapy and my passion. I've dealt with allergies all my life, so when I bought my bike I got a full face helmet. I thought that would protect me from the pollen 'soup' I ride through here in the local countryside. But a few weeks after getting my new bike I got my first sinus infection and they didn't stop - one right after the other.*

Now a sinus infection feels really icky, but not being able to ride because I was sick was just the pits.

I tried wearing a face mask to filter out particles. Talk about looking like a nerd on a Harley! The claustrophobia and the hassle factor didn't make me happy.

Finally I started to pack a travel-friendly nasal wash bottle in my saddlebags. And every time we stop for a break, I head for the bathroom or the bushes and discreetly wash my nose. You would not believe the stuff that comes out...just from riding! I know it's from the road because I wash my nose clean even before I get on the bike.

I've been riding without getting a sinus infection now for over a year. I still use my full face helmet, but no mask, and sometimes when the air smells sweet, I ride with the faceplate up just so I can enjoy the wind and the scents of the season. I don't know what I would have done without Nasopure. Thank you so much for giving me my passion back. **99**

Martha J., Lake County, California

SCORE!

66 I don't like taking any sort of drug. I tend to think 'by the time I take it and it takes effect, I'll feel better anyway.' Plus I really don't like the side effects of medication. The thing that I love about nasal washing is that it's pretty much instant relief with no side effects - except the relief! When you're all stuffed up, it feels SO GOOD to wash it out and then blow your nose and feel clear again. It feels like a SCORE when you get a Kleenex-full after a washing! As a runner and a cyclist, it's so valuable to be able to clear it all out when I'm a little (or a lot) stuffy so I can still get my workouts in. Or, during allergy season, coming home from a workout, hopping in the shower and washing out all of the gunk from being outside so I don't have to suffer later. **99**

Janna Sanders, Fitness Specialist Kansas City, Missouri

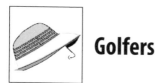 **Golfers**

Woman's Champion

66 *Anybody who spends time on a golf course knows that they inhale a considerable amount of irritants and pollutants - dirt, grit, sand, pollen, herbicides, and fertilizer - not to mention the germs and viruses one may encounter elsewhere. Nasal washing is the simplest, cheapest and most effective preventive regimen I've ever tried. Just by flushing your nose regularly you can prevent and relieve all kinds of nose-related annoyances and stay much healthier. In fact, I haven't gotten sick since I began using nasal washing last summer. No colds, no flu, no sinus troubles. So, it's great for golfers, but it works just as well for anyone who wants to keep their nose clean and their body healthy.* 99

Tree/Patricia Miller, Hartsburg, Missouri
2001 Eagle Knoll Women's Club Champion

Relief Achieved

66 *After four sinus surgeries and the constant sensation of stuffiness, I have achieved relief with nasal washing. I am able to walk on a golf course and breathe through my nose.* 99

Donald B, Doctor of Osteopathy
Muskegon, Michigan

Improved Performance

66 *I have been a runner all of my life. In fact, I earned a college scholarship because of my running. I have always suffered with allergies, beginning with allergy shots at an early age and almost daily medications. Then my boyfriend came home one day with a nose wash in hand and said, 'You have to try this' I was speechless as I stared at this crazy man! For starters, I had no idea what he was talking about, 'a nose wash?' Even after he showed me how to use it properly, it looked awkward and I had hesitations. He told me that washing my nasal passages would help my allergies and improve my performance as a runner. It was hard to turn something down that might help me succeed with my athletic career. I was also tired of taking antihistamines daily as well as antibiotics every few months. My nose was always stuffy, my head was always full. I told him that I would try it, only because I was desperate for some relief, so I was even willing to try this awkward weird new thing. The first time I used Nasopure was like nothing I had ever experienced. After daily washing for two weeks, I was actually amazed at how good I felt since I had been skeptical, to say the least. It did not cure my allergies, but it helped me breathe and breathing easier was a great thing. Because I am now able to breathe deeply and naturally, I can now focus on my running career. I am now medication-free, breathing deeper, and running harder.* **99**

Stefanie L, RN, University of Missouri
Columbia, Missouri

Hikers, Campers and Gardeners

 Being out in nature can lift your soul, but it can also congest your nasal passages. Anyone who spends time hiking in the great outdoors has a great reason to keep his or her nasal system clear and working properly. The same thing is true for people who spend a night (or a week or even more) sleeping under the stars. Remember also, that the harder you ask your body to work during your hikes, the more important it is for you to pay attention to the body's filter.

Congestion Clears Quickly

66 *I have found that often when I work in the yard at this time of year, I start sneezing and get congested. When I come inside, I do a nasal rinse and it is remarkable how the symptoms clear quickly. I was thinking that the habit of washing the nose should be similar to that of washing your hands. Make it part of personal hygiene.* **99**

Bob H, St Louis, Missouri

Scuba Divers

 Scuba divers need to equalize the pressure in their ears and sinuses, but they should not take medications immediately before diving. Nasal and/or sinus congestion can keep divers out of the water because of the pain caused by unequal ear pressure during the descent.

Some 30 years ago an expert in treatment of scuba divers, Los Angeles Ear, Nose and Throat specialist Dr. Murray Grossan, was led to the ancient practice of using salt water to rinse out the nose and sinuses. Dr. Grossan, a scuba diver himself, prescribed an updated version of that time-tested health practice. His patients rinsed with warm saline solution before diving to clear out their sinuses, allowing them to breathe freely and equalize pressure with few problems while underwater.

Healthy Habit

❝ *I start a regimen of daily use of nasal irrigation with buffered hypertonic nose washing for two weeks prior to any scuba diving trips I plan. Before I began this habit I had experienced painful dives if my nose was not absolutely clear. I cannot afford to plan a dive trip and then not be able to dive because I'm unable to equalize the pressure inside my ears when descending. So I have learned my lesson and use my nose wash to ensure that my Eustachian tubes are open, clean and working when it comes time to dive. It's simple, cheap, and easy-to-use insurance against possible cancellation of a dive.*

Glad my doctor suggested this common-sense approach. **❞**

George V. Z,
Hartsburg, Missouri

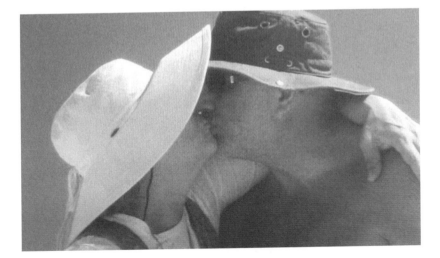

Conclusion

The idea of washing the body's filter, the nose, made sense to me the first time I was introduced to it decades ago. I incorporated this idea into my medical practice and witnessed, over the years, thousands of children and adults' health improved because they included nasal irrigation as part of their daily routine.

We have learned that brushing teeth prevents cavities. We wash hands to prevent the spread of germs. We shampoo our hair before it gets oily, greasy, and stinky. Cleaning the nose makes just as much sense as these other daily hygiene practices. With the overuse of antibiotics, the increase in drug resistance, and the move to more effective prevention, it's time we begin to care for our nose as often as we shower.

I understand this concept of nose washing is new to many people and yet millions around the world practice this technique daily. Have we become too comfortable taking pills? Or is nasal washing just too foreign an idea? My goal is to share my experience so you will consider cleaning before treating. Caring for your nose, just as you do all your other body parts will pay off. Take care of it and it will take care of you.

I sat in the audience of a Complementary and Alternative Medicine lecture presented by L. Bielory, MD during the 2006 American Academy of Allergy, Asthma and Immunology Conference. The original author is not known but he presented this slide, which I refer to often:

2000 B.C.E.: "Here, eat this root."

1000 C.E.: "That root is heathen. Here, say this prayer."

1850 C.E.: "That prayer is superstition. Here, drink this potion."

1940 C.E.: "That potion is snake oil. Here, swallow this pill."

1985 C.E.: "That pill is ineffective. Here, take this antibiotic."

2004 C.E.: "That antibiotic is artificial. Here, eat this root."

Perhaps in 2020 C.E. we will proudly state: medication use has dramatically decreased and is now taken with great respect. Antibiotic resistance has been eliminated through the drastic reduction in antibiotic use and abuse. Prevention is the new treatment goal for all medical providers.

I predict that nasal cleansing will become a vital part of daily hygiene for people in all cultures and walks of life around the globe. My husband, who continues to practice medicine from our home office, reminds his patients, "Pills can be poison. Take them only if you have no other options to solve your problems."

Be Well,

Dr. Hana

Hana R. Solomon, M.D.

Dr. Hana knowz Nozez

About the Author

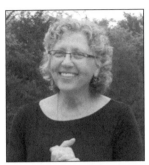

Hana R. Solomon, M.D. graduated from the University Of Missouri School Of Medicine in 1986 and was board certified in Pediatrics in 1989.

She and her husband, a physician, practiced medicine together in a mom and pop style clinic for 18 years.

Dr. Hana's focus on disease prevention and patient empowerment through education has always been her driving goal. She has been referenced in national publications such as Parents, Wall Street Journal, Health, and Alternative Medicine.

She lectures frequently to both medical and consumer audiences about preventative and natural approaches to nasal health issues. Devoted to her community as much as her practice, Dr. Hana has served as a sexual assault forensic examination physician, a volunteer board member for a home for abused and neglected children, and as a summer camp physician.

When she is not encouraging everyone to keep their noses clean, Dr. Hana enjoys gardening, pottery and being outdoors. She has four children and lives in Columbia, Missouri with her husband and best friend, George D. Solomon, M.D.

Contact Information: For information or permission to reproduce selections from this book, please contact Dr. Hana directly.

Hana R. Solomon, M.D.
573-999-0450
drhana@nasopure.com

References

1. Akinbami L; Schoendorf K: Trends in childhood asthma: prevalence, health care utilization, and mortality. PEDIATRICS Vol. 110 No. 2 August 2002, pp. 315-322.

2. Adams, P.,Hendershot, G:Current estimates from the National Health Interview Survey, 1996. Vital Health Statistics. 10(200).

3. Miller K; Siscovick D;,et al: Long-Term Exposure to Air Pollution and Incidence of Cardiovascular Events in Women. New England Journal of Medicine, Volume 356:447-458, February 1, 2007, Number 5.

4. Cisternas M; Blanc P; et al: A comprehensive study of the direct and indirect costs of adult asthma.¬† Journal of Allergy and Clinical Immunology, 2003,¬†Volume 111,¬†Issue 6,¬†Pages 1212 ,Äì 1218.

5. Ray N; Baraniuk J; Thamer M; et al: Healthcare expenditures for sinusitis in 1996: contributions or asthma, rhinitis and other airway disorders. Journal. of Allergy Clinical Immunology, 103 (3 Pt 1): 408-514, 1999.

6. Anand A, et al: Economic burden of rhinitis in managed care: a retrospective claims data analysis. Annals Allergy Asthma Immunology, 2008 Jul;101(1):23-9.

7. Monto A; Ullman B: Acute respiratory illness in an American community. Journal Of American Medical Association, 1974;227:164-169.

8. Bothwell M; Parsons D: Pediatric Chronic Rhinosinusitis: A Step-Wise Approach to Medical and Surgical Management. Operative Techniques in Otolaryngology - Head and Neck Surgery 12,1:34-39, 2001.

9. Rabago D; Zgierska A; et al: Efficacy of daily hypertonic saline irrigation among patients with sinusitis: a randomized controlled trial. Journal Family Practice 51(12): 1049-55, 2002 Dec.

10. Georgitis J.: Nasal Hyperthermia and Simple Irrigation for Perennial Rhinitis. Chest 106,5:1487-1491, 1994.

11. Grossan M: Irrigation of the Child,Äôs Nose. Clinical Pediatrics 13,3:229-231, 1974.

12. Grossan M: The Saccharin Test of Nasal Mucociliary Function. The Eye, Ear, Nose and Throat Monthly. 54:415-417, 1975.

13. Manning S: Pediatric Sinusitis. Otolaryngologic Clinics of North America. 26,4:623-637, 1993.

14. Rachelefsky G; Slavin R; Wald E: Sinusitis: Acute, Chronic - and Manageable. Patient Care. February 28, 1997 pp 105-117.

15. Salvin R; Cannon R; Friedman W: Sinusitis and Bronchial Asthma. Journal of Allergy and Clinical Immunology. 66,3:250-257, 1980.

16. Seaton T: Hypertonic Saline for Chronic Sinusitis. The Journal of Family Practice. 47,2:94-96.

17. Tomooka L; Murphy C; Davidson T: Clinical Study and Literature Review of Nasal Irrigation. The Laryngoscope. 110:1189-1192, 2000.

18. Virant F: A Guide to Therapeutic Interventions for Rhinosinusitis in Children. The Journal of Respiratory Diseases for Pediatricians . 4,1:8-14, 2002.

19. Zeiger R; Schatz   M: Chronic Rhinitis: A Practical Approach to Diagnosis and Treatment. Immunology & Allergy Practice. 4, 4:26-35.

20. Allergy and Asthma Center of Rochester, Michigan: Medical Conditions: Rhinitis and Pregnancy. Web site Jan 2003.

21. Shoseyov, D; Blbl H; et al: Treatment with hypertonic saline versus normal saline nasal wash of pediatric chronic sinusitis.¬† Journal of Allergy and Clinical Immunology 1998; 101:602-5.

22. Heatley D; McConnell K; et al: Nasal Irrigation for the alleviation of sinonasal symptoms. Presented at the annual Meeting of the American Academy of Otolaryngology- Head and Neck Surgery, Washington DC. 9/25/00.

23. Rabago D; Barrett B; Maberry R: Qualitative Aspects of Nasal Irrigation Use by Patients With Chronic Sinus Disease in a Multimethod Study. Annals of Family Medicine 4:295-301 (2006).

24. Sharp H; Denman D;Puumala S: Treatment of Acute and Chronic Rhinosinusitis in the United States, 1999-2002. Archives of Otolaryngology ,Äì Head & Neck Surgery 2007;133:260-265.

25. Harvey R; Hannan S; Badia L; Scadding G: Nasal saline irrigations for the symptoms of chronic rhinosinusitis. Cochrane Database System Review. 18;(3):CD006394. 2007.

26. Papsin B: Saline Nasal irrigation. Canadian Family Physician 49, 168-173, 2003.

27. Gonzales R; Malone D; Maselli J; Sande M: Excessive antibiotic use for acute respiratory infections in the United States. Clin Infect Dis. 2001;33:757-762.

28. American Lung Association.

29. Center for Disease Control.

30. National Institute of Health.

31. Current Allergy Asthma Report. 2002 May;2(3):223-30).

32. Prevention of Chronic Disease, 2005 Jan 2(1):A11.

33. National Center for Health Statistics. 1999.

34. Weiler JM, Bloomfield JR, Woodworth GG, Grant AR, Layton TA, Brown TL, McKenzie DR, Baker TW, Watson GS: Effects of fexofenadine, diphenhydramine, and alcohol on driving performance. Annals of Internal Medicine 2000 Mar 7; 132(5):354-63.

35. Bothwell MR, Parsons DS: Pediatric Chronic Rhinosinusitis: A step-wise approach to medical and surgical management. Operative Techniques in Otolaryngology-Head and Neck Surgery Vol 12(1), 34-39, 2001.

36. Pediatric Allergy Immunology 2003 Apr;14(2):140 in Pediatric Notes 2003 Jun 26;27(26):103.

37. Bailey B, ed. Nasal function and evaluation, nasal obstruction. Head and Neck Surgery: Otolaryngology. 2nd ed. New York, NY: Lippincott-Raven; 1998:335-44, 376, 380-90.

Index

A

Additives   *39, 40, 77, 78, 79, 84, 133*
Adenoids   *9, 46, 123, 129, 144, 206, 210, 213*
Ageusia   *22, 221–222*
Aging   *222, 227*
Airway   *14, 17, 19, 31, 41, 62, 77, 116, 143, 148, 151, 190, 195, 201, 204, 205, 207, 208, 219, 223, 224*
Allergic Rhinitis   *35, 62, 63, 149, 181, 184, 185, 186, 194, 227*
Allergy   *35, 56, 64, 146, 181, 183, 186, 205*
Alternative Medicine   *251*
Anosmia   *21, 222*
Antibiotics   *18, 39, 45, 46, 171, 180, 227*
Antihistamine   *42, 43, 44, 45, 56, 61, 76, 115, 128, 131, 143, 163, 166, 172, 179, 181, 213, 215, 218, 231, 236*
Anti-inflammatory   *155, 217*
Antimicrobials   *164*
Asthma   *19, 24, 35, 40, 44, 45, 51, 61, 62, 64, 87, 110, 116, 124, 125, 184, 186, 196, 201, 202, 203, 204, 209, 217, 251*
Athletes   *63, 243*

B

Babies   *1, 27, 121, 122, 123, 128, 224*
Bacteria   *15, 17, 18, 20, 31, 54, 61, 68, 70, 79, 80, 81, 83, 117, 171, 179, 180, 188, 191, 211, 213, 223, 225, 228*
Bacterial Infection   *18, 75, 79, 189*
Bad Breath   *15, 63, 68, 171, 213*
Barberry (Berberis Vulgaris)   *82*
Berberine Botanicals   *82*
Bernoulli's Principle   *100, 101*
Biofilm   *70, 80, 81, 171*
Bleeding   *46, 180, 214, 216*
Body Odor   *23, 222*

Bronchial Dilator   *45*
Bronchial Tubes   *19, 204*
Bronchitis   *44, 51, 152, 158, 198, 241, 242*
Bronchospasm   *209*
Buffering   *33, 71, 84, 104, 112*

C

Caffeine   *148, 162, 197*
Cardiovascular   *150*
Chemotherapy   *37, 39*
Children   *2, 16, 22, 30, 35, 36, 40, 42, 43, 44, 51, 73, 75, 76, 81, 85, 92, 97, 105, 109, 116, 125, 127, 128, 129, 131, 132, 133, 136, 137, 138, 142, 144, 146, 157, 160, 161, 162, 164, 167, 168, 169, 181, 185, 186, 190, 191, 196, 201, 202, 205, 206, 210, 213, 215, 226, 227, 237, 251*
Chronic Illness   *170, 181, 185, 186*
Chronic Inflammatory Disease   *201*
Chronic Nasal Congestion   *128*
Chronic Sinusitis   *170, 171, 173, 179, 180*
Cilia   *15, 16, 17, 19, 20, 26, 27, 33, 100, 161, 179, 186, 223, 224, 240*
Common Cold   *18, 41, 61, 68, 150, 157, 158, 159, 160, 161, 165, 167, 188, 222*
Congestion   *16, 26, 39, 40, 41, 57, 61, 64, 76, 84, 89, 91, 99, 108, 116, 128, 129, 142, 147, 148, 149, 151, 152, 163, 165, 166, 169, 181, 183, 184, 187, 190, 194, 195, 200, 204, 208, 210, 212, 218, 222, 223, 235, 242, 248*
COPD (chronic obstructive pulmonary disease)   *196*
Cough   *1, 17, 18, 44, 51, 62, 114, 124, 127, 142, 144, 145, 152, 155, 157, 158, 161, 169, 189, 192, 195, 196, 198, 199, 200*

CPAP   *63, 64, 148, 207, 208*
Croup   *196*
Cystic Fibrosis   *51, 62, 63, 217, 218, 224, 225, 226, 227*

D

Decongestant   *40, 41, 42, 43, 56, 61, 110, 127, 132, 148, 161, 163, 166, 172, 205, 236, 239*
Deviated Septum   *28, 91, 207, 219, 221*
Dry Mouth   *43, 213*

E

Ear   *3, 5, 8, 9, 17, 18, 24, 29, 30, 31, 33, 35, 41, 55, 64, 67, 72, 87, 91, 92, 97, 108, 110, 111, 124, 125, 127, 128, 129, 131, 133, 142, 143, 144, 147, 154, 158, 162, 166, 193, 196, 209, 210, 211, 212, 233, 248*
Ear Canal   *29, 129, 193, 210, 233*
Ear Drum   *9, 143*
Ear Infections   *5, 18, 31, 35, 54, 62, 79, 125, 128, 129, 131, 142, 158, 162, 196, 209, 210, 211*
Ear Wax   *29*
Environment   *3, 7, 13, 15, 18, 23, 25, 28, 37, 51, 52, 54, 63, 72, 123, 131, 161, 182, 185, 200, 210, 213, 224, 235, 241, 242*
Epistaxis   *214, 216*
Eustachian Tube   *9, 17, 30, 31, 76, 79, 111, 128, 129, 154, 209, 210, 211, 249*
Eyes   *24, 32, 42, 43, 51, 83, 107, 136, 139, 144, 154, 163, 171, 184, 234, 241*

F

Facial Pressure   *147, 152*
Facts   *33*
Flu   *15, 64, 114, 127, 157, 158, 159, 161, 165, 169, 200, 246*
Fungal Spores   *179*

G

Gastroesophageal Reflux   *123, 131, 195*
Goldenseal (Hydrastis canadensis)   *82*

Golfers   *246*

H

Halitosis   *213*
Hay Fever   *35, 41, 181, 194, 232*
Headache   *1, 15, 17, 24, 42, 47, 51, 157, 159, 166, 171, 172, 190, 217, 219*
Hearing Problems   *209*
Heart Disease   *150*
Hikers   *248*
Histamines   *42, 82*
Hormones   *17, 147, 194*
Humidity   *151, 162, 163, 200*
Hydration   *17, 131, 224*
Hypertension   *42, 208*
Hypertonic   *26, 33, 42, 57, 65, 67, 68, 69, 70, 72, 73, 74, 75, 76, 77, 82, 83, 84, 89, 92, 95, 106, 108, 111, 112, 113, 115, 130, 133, 144, 146, 148, 152, 159, 172, 178, 181, 193, 195, 200, 218, 219, 224, 229, 236, 249*
Hypotonic   *67, 70*

I

Immotile Cilia   *223, 224*
Infants   *33, 37, 121, 123, 127, 128, 142, 162, 184, 196*
Infection   *5, 17, 18, 19, 20, 28, 29, 31, 33, 35, 41, 43, 45, 46, 47, 51, 54, 61, 62, 64, 68, 69, 74, 75, 77, 79, 80, 83, 87, 98, 109, 123, 142, 153, 158, 163, 165, 167, 173, 174, 175, 178, 179, 187, 188, 189, 191, 205, 207, 210, 211, 212, 222, 224, 225, 226, 228, 229, 240, 244, 245*
Inflammation   *21, 41, 46, 72, 82, 83, 110, 170, 176, 179, 184, 185, 189, 192, 201, 210, 216, 218, 221*
Influenza   *157, 158, 159, 162, 200*
Isotonic   *33, 67, 69, 70, 72, 84, 106, 108, 112, 113, 115, 123, 133, 138*

K

Kids and Colds   *127*
Kiesselbach's area   *214*

M

Middle ear   *128, 129, 142, 144, 209, 210, 211, 233*
Military   *237*
Molds   *19, 179*
Mononucleosis   *188*
MRSA   *47, 74, 178, 228, 229*
Mucolytics   *43, 44, 45, 161*

N

Nasopure   *7, 47, 59, 91, 92, 95, 99, 100, 101, 103, 104, 105, 106, 110, 114, 116, 118, 134, 143, 153, 166, 172, 174, 198, 199, 226, 227, 234, 235, 236, 238, 239, 245, 247*
Nasopure Effect   *100*
Nose Bleed   *62, 99, 214, 219*

O

Obstructive Sleep Apnea   *208, 218*
Otitis Media   *211, 212*
Outer Ear Infection   *210*

P

Pollen   *19, 20, 21, 32, 42, 76, 92, 115, 179, 181, 182, 183, 184, 185, 186, 187, 194, 199, 203, 205, 221, 235, 244, 246*
Pollution   *15, 17, 19, 51, 52, 53, 87, 116, 128, 150, 194, 201, 203, 241*
Polyps   *51, 91, 171, 179, 184, 186, 207, 216, 217, 218, 221, 222, 224, 225, 233*
Popping   *87, 111, 152, 209*
Post Nasal Drip   *62, 159, 198*
Pregnancy   *26, 62, 63, 147, 148, 149, 215*
Preschoolers   *164*
Prevention   *2, 36, 39, 54, 55, 63, 64, 75, 109, 113, 133, 157, 159, 187, 201, 229, 251, 252*
Primary Ciliary Dyskinesia   *223*
Proetz Procedure   *55*
Pseudomonas Aeruginosa   *80*

Q

Quercetin   *82*

R

Rebound Nasal Congestion   *40*
References   *255*
Resistant Bacteria   *180, 228*
Rhinitis   *16, 35, 40, 62, 63, 147, 148, 149, 163, 181, 184, 185, 186, 192, 194, 195, 215, 227*
Rhinovirus   *160*

S

Scarlet Fever   *190*
Scleroderma   *55*
scuba diving   *249*
Sexuality   *23*
Singers   *233*
Sinus   *3, 5, 7, 9, 15, 16, 17, 18, 19, 25, 26, 27, 28, 33, 35, 41, 43, 45, 46, 55, 56, 61, 62, 63, 64, 67, 73, 79, 80, 83, 84, 85, 91, 92, 94, 95, 101, 103, 108, 110, 111, 114, 116, 118, 124, 127, 133, 134, 144, 147, 152, 153, 154, 155, 158, 162, 165, 166, 168, 169, 170, 171, 172, 173, 174, 175, 176, 177, 178, 179, 180, 185, 186, 187, 188, 189, 190, 195, 196, 203, 204, 205, 207, 208, 209, 210, 213, 217, 218, 221, 222, 223, 224, 225, 226, 227, 228, 229, 231, 233, 235, 236, 239, 242, 244, 245, 246, 248*
Sinusitis   *18, 35, 41, 46, 56, 62, 72, 80, 82, 92, 116, 170, 171, 172, 173, 174, 178, 179, 180, 184, 185, 186, 196, 215, 217, 222, 227, 233*
Sleep   *17, 35, 42, 43, 44, 63, 64, 117, 124, 125, 147, 149, 152, 162, 183, 188, 195, 206, 207, 208, 217, 218, 221*
Sleep Apnea   *63, 64, 207, 208, 217, 218*
Smell   *15, 17, 21, 22, 23, 28, 47, 52, 61, 63, 64, 68, 148, 149, 151, 189, 217, 221, 222, 223*
Smokers   *65, 240*
Sneezing   *147, 154, 167, 181, 184, 200, 248*
Snoring   *1, 24, 62, 63, 117, 147, 206, 207, 208, 217, 225*
Sports   *209, 243*
Staphylococcus Aureus   *228*

Steroids   *100, 116, 148, 179, 201, 204,*
          205, 218, 233
Strep   *188, 189, 190, 191*
Swimmers Ear   *210, 211*

T

Taste   *15, 17, 21, 22, 24, 33, 62, 63, 64,*
          88, 107, 124, 151, 189, 193, 196,
          221, 222, 223
Throat   *1, 3, 8, 14, 15, 17, 19, 24, 25, 30,*
          31, 51, 55, 62, 64, 72, 73, 74, 76, 79,
          88, 90, 97, 107, 109, 110, 111, 113,
          115, 124, 128, 129, 133, 143, 144,
          152, 153, 154, 155, 157, 161, 171,
          172, 180, 188, 189, 190, 191, 192,
          193, 195, 196, 197, 203, 207, 208,
          209, 210, 212, 213, 214, 215, 224,
          226, 233, 241, 248
Thrombocytopenia   *215*
Toddlers   *136*
Tonsil   *129, 143, 189, 190, 213*
Tonsillitis   *189, 190*
Toxic Mold   *180*
Traveling   *235, 238, 239*
Triggers   *171, 201, 202, 203*

V

Vasomotor Rhinitis   *194, 195*
Viral Infection   *123, 127, 157, 202*
Vocal Cord   *196, 233*

W

Women   *2, 17, 42, 147, 148, 149, 150,*
          169, 194, 246